Alternative Conception

From Infertility to Delivery

Dr. Mimi Amaral, PSY.D.

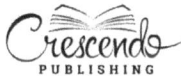

Crescendo
PUBLISHING

Alternative Conception: From Infertility to Delivery
Copyright © 2021 by Dr. Mimi Amaral, PSY.D.

Crescendo Publishing, LLC
2-558 Upper Gage Ave., Ste. 246
Hamilton, ON L8V 4J6
Canada

GetPublished@CrescendoPublishing.com
1-877-575-8814

ISBN: 978-1-948719-33-9
ISBN: 978-1-948719-34-6

Printed in the United States of America
Cover Design by Nouman Sarwar
Original Cover Art by Dr. Mimi Amaral

10 9 8 7 6 5 4 3 2 1

IVF can be a daunting journey for most, and trying to understand everything that goes into each step can create anxiety. The aspiration of this book is to be a reference to help ease the stress of the journey by outlining as much information as possible.

Message from the Author

First, acknowledgment and gratitude to cosmic alignment and divine guidance (AKA: Source/ Universe/God).

I have never claimed to have all the answers because I do not. All I can say is that I can hold a safe space to toss ideas around so a co-creation of answers may be manifested.

In this book, I tried to outline as many infertility issues as possible and aspects of IVF that may occur along the journey to having a family. In addition, I came from a perspective of experience. I have personally embraced the infertility and IVF journey. I did my best to remain mindful and neutral while collecting information on as many subjects that may come up during the pre-decision phase through the delivery of child/children.

Topics covered but are not limited to conception struggles, infertility, mental and emotional wellness, introduction to IVF, IVF options, the IVF doctor process, medication, procedures, agency, and surrogacy, transfer to implant, and transition to OB/ GYN.

Dedications

This book was written with the aspiration to empower intended parent(s) with as much information as possible to ease the whirlwind of uncertainty and questioning surrounding infertility and In-Vitro Fertilization (IVF). Furthermore, it has been created to guide the reader through the options and process of the IVF journey.

I aspire for this book to help all who may take the alternative conception process toward creating and/or expanding their family.

Disclaimer

Always consult with your physician(s) throughout the IVF process and continue to communicate everything you are doing. This includes, but is not limited to, nutritional regimens, vitamin and supplement regimens, and medications, as well as your emotional, mental, and physical states.

This book is simply a collection of information with the aim to inform and help with the journey of infertility and IVF. Everyone's journey may be different and complex in their own way because every human's biology—physical, emotional, and mental—is unique.

Additionally, the information implemented within this book is for the sole purpose of giving a realistic view of current information. It is not to promote or endorse any process, doctor, lawyer, insurance, or facility. Always research all doctors, lawyers, insurance, facilities, clinics, medications, and any other variables that may coincide with each individual journey. It is best for each couple to understand all aspects of their own process and make informed decisions for their unique situation.

Foreword

By
Dr. T. Owens-Gager, EdD
Psychologist

Regardless of culture, race, or social status, giving birth and beginning a family is a happy occasion. This is especially true of a first child. Almost every culture has some type of birth ritual as a result. But what happens when a couple cannot conceive? For some, the pressure to provide a child for their partner or family is so intense that it becomes a struggle fraught with depression and anxiety. If this is the case, a mental health professional should be included as part of the fertility treatment.

The United States is a developed nation that is experiencing a population increase, while most developed nations are experiencing fewer births and expect population decreases over the next 50 years. For the most part, people living in developed nations do not need large families, but the United States still has a high fertility rate. The population of the U.S. is currently at approximately 330 million. By 2060, that number is expected to be 447 million people. There are a few reasons for this. One is that the U.S. allows more immigration than any other developed nation. Another is that the total fertility rate of the U.S. is around 2.0, meaning there is an average of approximately 2 births per woman of childbearing years.

Other developed nations such as Finland and Norway are experiencing declines in the fertility rate at 1.4 and 1.6, respectively. Alternatively, developing nations such as Kenya (3.5) and Nigeria (5.4) are holding steady with their relatively high fertility rates. The reasons the U.S. may be experiencing a higher fertility rate are partly due to the high number of people holding religious beliefs. These belief systems tend to focus on, and value, families. While there are several beliefs that can impact the desire for children, religion is one of the biggest.

Being unable to have children can put couples in a cycle of trying, hoping, experiencing sadness, and grasping for any possibility of giving birth. While the U.S. uses a science-based approach to fertility treatment, any prenatal belief is impacted by the generational wisdom of the time. Currently, couples can use drug-based fertility treatments, artificial insemination, In-Vitro Fertilization, and surrogacy. Many historic beliefs included:

- Avoiding wine
- Specific types of meat
- Certain types of hot, cold food
- Witches
- Strong foods

Once a couple conceives, the focus shifts from the struggle of conception to the fear and wariness that the pregnancy may be too good to be true. This anxiety is common and eases over the duration of the pregnancy. Some current science-driven prenatal methods are derived from traditional methods which include massages, exercise, diet, and avoiding any teratogen.

Once the prenatal process is complete and it is time to deliver the neonate, there are three stages. The first stage, labor, is the longest and most taxing stage, where contractions in the uterus cause the cervix to dilate. Labor is painful, but there are ways to ease the discomfort, if only a little. Sitting in a rocking chair, taking a warm shower or bath, getting massages, or taking a walk can all help. The single most important factor in easing the labor process is emotional support. Emotional support is also extremely important while trying to conceive. Stress hormones cause harm to the body, and having appropriate emotional support eases the strain of trying to conceive.

The second stage, birth and delivery, can take up to an hour after the initial hours of labor, wherein support and care are very important. After the neonate is born, the umbilical cord and placenta (afterbirth) are delivered. It is important that a qualified individual assists during this process. Complications could occur if the placenta is not fully expelled, and sometimes a complication is as simple as an adverse emotional reaction. The overwhelming emotions during childbirth can trigger the release of epinephrine and cease the release of oxytocin, which halts the birth process.

Once the child is born, a couple or individual who initially had difficulty with conception may still feel anxious or depressed, but the feelings connected with the struggle to conceive may fade over time. If those feelings do not fade, it is important to speak to a mental health professional.

It is very important to note that the feelings of anxiety, pressure, stress, and depression can be present in both partners, not just the one designated to conceive. Both partners, either in a same-sex or opposite-sex couple, can experience these emotions as well as postpartum depression. It is important to utilize the resources available, a discussion of which is found throughout this book.

Table of Contents

Foreword.. xi

Chapter 1 Struggling to Conceive 1
Chapter 2 Stress and Wellness 19
Chapter 3 Introduction to Conception and IVF 41
Chapter 4 Transfer to OB/GYN..61
Chapter 5 IVF Cost 83

About the Author.. 99
Other Books by Mimi Amaral 101
Connect with the Author 103
Acknowledgements..105
With Special Gratitude..107
References 109

Chapter 1

Struggling to Conceive

When an opposite-sex couple is trying to start their family, an in-depth conversation around conception and the potential of infertility does not often come to play. Instead, the joy from the idea of creating life is usually the focus. However, once a couple has been trying for a while and nothing happens, concerns and questions begin to form. Though it is not an everyday conversation in most cultures, this discussion is not uncommon for couples who struggle with conception and infertility.

Same-sex couples who aspire to create their family may find the conversation surrounding conception to be a more common occurrence in their journey. Additionally, same-sex couples can also struggle during the process of creating a family, and if conception for either same-sex male(s) or female(s) occurs, much of the following information may be beneficial.

The Center for Disease Control (CDC) has stated, "About 6% of married women aged 15 to 44 years in the United States are unable to get pregnant after one year of trying (infertility). Also, about 12% of women 15 to 44 years in the United States have difficulty getting pregnant or carrying a pregnancy to term, regardless of marital status (impaired fecundity)." Additionally, Resolve indicated, "A couple ages 29-33 with a normal functioning reproductive system has only a 20-25% chance of conceiving in any given month."

No one wants to acknowledge the possibility of conception issue within their own family. However, there may be many reasons for conception or infertility, and both women and men may contribute to the biological difficulty and lack of pregnancy. In fact, the McFarland Clinic indicated, "There are a wide variety of causes of infertility in both men and women, which is why working with your physician on the appropriate infertility testing is important."

Finding the cause

After a year of unsuccessfully trying to get pregnant, a couple may want to consult their doctor. However, if there is a family history of difficulty conceiving, a couple may want to consult with their general practitioner sooner. Thereafter the couple's doctor can refer them to a specialist who may begin specific tests.

At this point, a couple may be recommended to an obstetrician to discuss infertility and the potential causes. Once this discussion occurs, fertility testing is usually recommended to pinpoint any underlining issues. As indicated by McFarland Clinic, "A typical infertility work-up at a clinic may include BBT (basal body temperature), charting, blood tests, an ultrasound, a hysterosalpingogram (HSG), semen analysis, and sometimes diagnostic laparoscopy."

Infertility

Many think that infertility is simply the inability to conceive a child. However, there is a lot more that goes into the concept and reality of infertility and the lack of conception. As described by NHS, "Infertility is when a couple cannot get pregnant (conceive) despite having regular unprotected sex, and infertility is usually only diagnosed when a couple has not managed to conceive after a year of trying." Whereas Very Well Family stated, "Infertility refers to how long you have been trying to conceive unsuccessfully. While there are possible early warning signs of infertility as well as risk factors some couples don't have any signs or symptoms of infertility."

This sounds basic enough, and precisely what one would think when hearing the word "infertility." But with all complicated subjects, it goes much deeper than the surface layer and concept above. In fact, NHS described two types of infertility:

- Primary Infertility: Where someone who has never conceived a child in the past has difficulty in conceiving.
- Secondary Infertility: Where someone has had one or more pregnancies in the past but is having difficulty conceiving again.

The two types are what may be described as a deeper level of infertility. But, again, the layers go even deeper. For example, there are many causes and risk factors that can contribute to infertility. The Cleveland Clinic explains that infertility can occur for many reasons, but four things need to happen for a couple to become pregnant, including:

- A woman must produce and release a healthy egg from one of her ovaries (ovulation).
- A man must produce viable sperm which can successfully fertilize the woman's egg (fertilization).
- The egg must travel through a fallopian tube toward the uterus (transportation).

- The fertilized egg must attach to the inside of the uterus (implantation).

In addition, Cleveland Clinic stated that the issues creating infertility may manifest through "[p]roblems with egg or sperm production, genetic factors, age, or too much exposure to certain chemicals or toxins." The depth and breadth of conception and infertility are much more complex than is truly discussed within many cultures. In fact, if the above was not enough to think about, NHS has outlined some risk factors that also contribute to infertility. The following is not an exhaustive list, but rather a few variables that may contribute to infertility:

- Age: Fertility declines with age.
- Weight: Being overweight or obese reduces fertility in women (having a BMI of 30 or over).
- Sexually transmitted infection (STIs): Several STIs, including Chlamydia, can affect fertility.
- Smoking: Affects chance of conceiving and can reduce semen quality.
- Alcohol: The safest approach is to not drink alcohol at all to keep risk to the baby at a minimum. Drinking too much alcohol can also reduce quality of sperm.

- Environment Factors: Exposure to certain pesticides, solvents, and metals has been shown to affect fertility, particularly in men.
- Stress: Can affect your relationship with your partner and cause a loss of sex drive; in severe cases, stress may also affect ovulation and sperm production.

Another aspect not mentioned above is pre-existing medical conditions. Conception and infertility consist of more variables than most may consider. Again, the problems do not rest solely on the female; it is true that males can also have fertility issues.

If I may suggest taking a minute to exhale here and digest the information thus far, it may be beneficial.

To better understand some of the more specific individual concerns for each couple, female and male causes and/or symptoms are referenced by the Mayo Clinic:

Female Fertility Issues

For females, possible obvious indications of conception or infertility issues may be irregular or missed menstrual cycles. With such symptoms, following up with a doctor for the cause is recommended. The Mayo

Clinic detailed a few causes that may contribute to female reproductive issues:

- Ovulation disorders: these disorders affect the release of eggs from the ovaries. These include hormonal disorders such as polycystic ovary syndrome.
- Hyperprolactinemia: a condition in which you have too much prolactin—the hormone that stimulates breast milk production—and may also interfere with ovulation.
- Uterine or cervical abnormalities: this includes abnormalities with the cervix, polyps in the uterus, or the shape of the uterus.
- Uterine fibroids: these benign (noncancerous) tumors in the uterine wall may cause infertility by blocking the fallopian tubes or stopping a fertilized egg from implanting in the uterus.
- Fallopian tube damage: blockage often caused by inflammation of the fallopian tube (salpingitis).
- Endometriosis: a disorder that occurs when endometrial tissue grows outside of the uterus and may affect the function of the ovaries, uterus, and fallopian tubes.

- Primary Ovarian Insufficiency: sometimes called early menopause, when the ovaries stop working and menstruation ends before age 40.
- Pelvic adhesions: bands of scar tissue that bind organs and can form after pelvic infection, appendicitis, endometriosis, or abdominal or pelvic surgery.

According to the Mayo Clinic, these variables are only a few female reproductive complications. Again, these are only one partner's contribution. The male, or second partner, may also have fertility complications.

Male Fertility Issues

Nobody is immune to fertility issues, including men. As indicated by the Mayo Clinic, some reproductive concerns for males may include the following:

- Abnormal sperm production or function due to undescended testicles, genetic defects, health problems such as diabetes, or infections such as Chlamydia, gonorrhea, mumps, or HIV.
- Problems with the delivery of sperm due to sexual problems such as premature ejaculation; genetic diseases such as cystic fibrosis, or structural problems.
- Overexposure to certain environmental factors such as pesticides and other chemicals, radia-

tion, cigarette smoking, alcohol, marijuana, anabolic steroids, and taking medications to treat bacterial infections.

Again, these are merely a few examples that the Mayo Clinic indicated for male infertility. There are many reasons infertility in males can occur; therefore, it is best to consult with a doctor as soon as the concern for infertility has been recognized.

Miscarriage

The occurrence of a miscarriage is more common than one would think, yet there seem to be few healthy conversations around this subject. In fact, many women may feel isolated if a miscarriage occurs and fearful to reach out to tell a family member or a friend.

Katherine Martinelli, who wrote an article discussing the subject of miscarriage, interviewed a woman named Krista Gervan who miscarried at seven weeks. Gervan openly shared her experience of miscarriage with other women and was surprised by how many women opened up and talked about their experiences.

Within the interview, Gervan disclosed she is co-producing, with filmmaker Ann Zamudio, a documentary titled *Don't Talk About the Baby*. Gervan stated, "We want to break the stigma and silence around infertility and pregnancy loss. We want it to be something people talk about openly and not feel like it's something to be ashamed of or embarrassed by or that it is something wrong with them."

At this point, a couple may wonder about the frequency of a miscarriage. The American Pregnancy Association indicated, "Studies reveal that anywhere from 10-25% of all clinically recognized pregnancies will end in miscarriage. Chemical pregnancies may account for 50-75% of all miscarriages." With such a high percentage, one may wonder why this subject is not openly discussed. Furthermore, the chances of having a miscarriage, outlined by the American Pregnancy Association, are as follows:

- Women under the age of 35 years old have about a 15% chance of miscarriage.
- An increase in maternal age affects the chances of miscarriage.
- Women who are 35 to 45 years old have a 20 to 35% chance of miscarriage.
- Women over the age of 45 years can have up to 50% chance of miscarriage.
- A woman who has had a previous miscarriage has a 25% chance of having another.

Reviewing the data, it may seem bewildering to think that a topic that has such high statistical occurrence is not openly discussed. Other factors may contribute to miscarriage, and there are multiple types of miscarriage

ALTERNATIVE CONCEPTION

and related issues that can be further researched if one wishes to do their due diligence on this subject.

Lastly are the myths regarding infertility tossed about throughout the ages. Many have heard the superstitions or myths of infertility, and some may have even been given "advice" on how to rectify the situation. The following are some inaccurate perceptions of infertility.

Myths

Looking at some misconceptions that surround infertility can be beneficial. False thoughts, or myths, can come about and create undue stress, and below is a glimpse at seven myths shared by the online resource, *Parents*.

Myth	Fact
It's easy for most women to get pregnant	Though it is true many women conceive without difficulty, more than 5 million people of childbearing age in the United States have problems with infertility.
Men do not have fertility problems.	Though it's commonly believed that infertility is a "women's problem" nothing is further from the truth. About 35 percent of all fertility issues in the United States are due to female problems. But 35 percent (an equal number) can be traced to male problems.
Infertility is a Psychological – Not Physical – problem.	Well-meaning friends or relatives may suggest "infertility is all in your head" or "If you stop worrying so much, you'd get pregnant." But in reality, infertility is a disease or condition of the reproductive system, and not a psychological disorder.
Couples who "work" hard enough at having a baby will eventually get pregnant.	According to American Society for Reproductive Medicine (ASRM), more than half of all couples who pursue treatment will achieve a successful pregnancy. On the other hand, it is important to remember that infertility is a medical disease and that problems sometimes remain untreatable
Once a couple adopts a child, the woman will become pregnant.	This statement suggests that adoption is simply a means to an end (pregnancy), and not a valid and wonderful way to form a family. Only about 5% of couples who adopt later become pregnant.
Husbands often leave their wives if they're infertile.	While many couples do find the process of infertility testing and treatment rigorous, stressful, and intrusive (not to mention costly), they do get through it – together. Many partners also find new and deeper ways of relating to each other and discover that their marriage has become even stronger.
Infertile couples will never be happy or fulfilled.	Being unable to conceive a much-wanted child (or carry a pregnancy to term) can fill a couple with sadness, grief, anger, despair, and even a sense of personal failure. While its normal for infertile couples to experience a range of emotions, most people do move through this life crisis successfully and gradually put it into better perspective.

Many of us may have heard some of the above myths and internalized them without knowing. It is amazing how misconception of a topic may potentially hinder the entire process. By outlining some of these myths, we may help ease the misinformation.

Testimonials

Feeling paralyzed (Male)

As a man, it's hard for me to know exactly what to say or do when facing potential infertility. Especially seeing how the struggle affects my partner.

I try to comfort her as best I can, and often I feel inadequate that I can't just make this issue go away, like any man would want to do, by fixing something that's bothering the woman he loves.

I've wondered, as she went to appointments getting tests and feeling frustrated every month as she tested negative, if it was me causing the issues and how me and my lifestyle might have impacted this journey.

I've felt guilty about if maybe I stressed her too much in the past with my own issues and that's why she wasn't easily getting pregnant or able to carry full term now.

I do really want to have a child with my partner, and it's hard seeing her disappointment each month that we struggle with fertility. I'm still hopeful and confident that we will be able to conceive and carry successfully and have a beautiful healthy baby together, despite the struggles we have faced.

We are fully committed to being successful in this together, and I really can't wait to see the physical manifestation of our love in an awesome little human.

Failed Attempts (Female)

My journey has been one of confusion, disappointment, dashed hopes, negative tests month after month, blaming myself, and feeling incapable as a woman. It's not something I talk about or share often, as it can be embarrassing and elicit unwanted judgment.

I've tried the spiritual route, the medical route, and finally just leaving it up to chance. I even go through cycles where I question if I even want another baby anymore, but I always come back to the desire in my heart to bring forth another awesome human being. There are months I've felt hopeful, and months I just assumed failure and didn't even bother hoping. So many times, I just knew I was pregnant only to have the pregnancy test tell me otherwise. Each time was a huge letdown.

I quickly tried to encourage myself through those moments and say "next month for sure." I queued up my cycle tracker, made sure I was ovulating, and followed suggestions from women on online forums (sic) who had been trying for years and were finally successful. I do have an older child whom I didn't struggle with conceiving at all, but that was nearly 15 years ago.

In my new relationship, my hope was that we would have a healthy child together. After being unsuccessful in having a healthy pregnancy after 5 years together, I have grown weary but not lost hope. I sought medical intervention for about 4 years. Thus far, no medical cause has been uncovered, but I will say I'm quite sure that stress has been a factor in my infertility.

My focus now is on becoming as spiritually aligned as possible with welcoming a child into my womb to stay and grow healthy and be born into our family with no complications. I still pray, I still am doing what I can to manifest our rainbow miracle baby into our lives and staying hopeful and open to new solutions. Though this journey can be painful and sad, I know God is still in the miracle-making business and anything is possible. I have hope.

First Miscarriage

I remember the day of my friend's party. Knowing at any time I could be passing my dead baby through me... just waiting for the process to begin. The day before, I had been at my first doctor's visit for my first pregnancy and had received the bad news.

I was so excited to see the baby, but when they did the ultrasound, they saw nothing. The baby had disappeared.

They told me I would either miscarry naturally or I was having an ectopic pregnancy and would need surgery and might not be able to have a normal pregnancy ever.

I left the appointment sad, scared, and stunned. I felt numb. When I had found out I was pregnant I went through a range of emotions starting with scared then eventually feeling excited thinking about names and the future.

The strange thing about a miscarriage is you almost feel robbed. Robbed of what could have been, tossed in with a bit of guilt, sprinkled with shame.

You ask, "Why me? Is my body bad, did I do something wrong?" You rethink everything over and over in your head. It can drive you crazy wondering how it happened. Then, you suffer the loss of what your imagination had planned for the future and you also feel embarrassed. You don't really feel adequate and wonder if you will be judged by others as a failure. I think this is why most women keep silent. I told only a handful of people.

So back to the party... Why was I at a party when I am supposed to be sad? I wanted to have a sense of normalcy and get my mind off the situation, so I went as a distraction. Once I was there, the heavy bleeding and cramps started. I asked my husband to drive me home. He wanted to stay with me and comfort me, but I really wanted to be alone and unbothered. I sat alone in my bed, bleeding, cramping, back and forth to the toilet waiting for the mess to be over with. I knew it would never be out of my mind even if my body would heal.

Looking back, I am glad I let myself have the alone "me" time. It was healing to sit alone in my sorrow and feel the pain and sadness. I also had a doctor call me to check in, and she was so compassionate and let me know she too had miscarried, and it was okay. I'll never forget her kindness.

Moving forward to present time, I am now a mom to two healthy girls. I was fearful each pregnancy of another miscarriage but was lucky to have healthy pregnancies both times. They say 1 of 3 of pregnancies end in miscarriage, and that was me exactly; 1 out of 3.

Time heals all, as they say, but the feeling of losing what could have been sticks with you. You learn to accept it and move forward, but it's never forgotten and is always a part of your story. It places you among many other women who are warriors, who have been through the same situation and the many more to follow. You can use your own story to ease the pain for others. This is what I have done and will continue to do.

Chapter 2

Stress and Wellness

Just like any major transition or milestone in life, some stress may accompany the process of alternative fertilization. It is best to keep in mind that there is a spectrum to everything, including how everyone may process the journey. Some couples may decide to try for a limited time due to finances or to minimize emotional, mental, and physical hardship, while other couples may decide that there is no limit, and the end process is to produce a child.

Once a couple realizes they will need help to conceive, it may be best to take the time to discuss the parameters and financial allowance that are safely feasible to manifest the desired outcome. It is also wise to make a plan B that outlines how to support one another after the established agreed-upon process has been reached, should pregnancy not occur.

After processing that natural conception is not possible and help will be needed, emotions may induce an internal rumination leading to an increase in stress hormones, which may also contribute to the issues of infertility. Understanding how stress may contribute to infertility is important.

Conception Stress

The concept that stress may potentially contribute to infertility has been a topic discussed for many decades. As described by Amos Grunebaum, "When a couple tries to conceive, problems with infertility can lead to stress. Stress has a physical and emotional effect on both partners which can impede fertility both physically and mentally. Physically the body can release increased amounts of hormones as a natural reaction to stress. Mentally, stress factors can cause erectile dysfunction and a lack of interest in sex."

Various types of stress may occur during the alternative fertility route, and each may contribute to the problem in unique ways. As indicated by Hallie Levine, "Several recent studies have found links between the women's levels of day-to-day stress and lowered chances of pregnancy. For example, women whose saliva had high levels of alpha-amylase, an enzyme that makes stress, took 29% longer to get pregnant compared to those who had less."

Mental and physical stress processes have been briefly mentioned above. However, emotional stress can also be a contributing factor, which may be experienced on a spectrum depending on a person's subjective perspective of the journey.

Alternative Reproduction Stress

Trying to conceive naturally may be stressful in and of itself, but when the variables of infertility, doctors, tests, medications, and more are tossed into the mix, it can feel like a rollercoaster ride. As described by Southern California Reproductive Center, "Infertility can take an emotional toll on women and couples. Disappointment and heartbreak may go on for years, and by the time a patient seeks out fertility treatment their emotional reserves may be very low."

Many couples may even experience a level of uncertainty and/or anxiety surrounding the process of treatments. Let us take In-Vitro Fertilization (IVF), for example; there are many steps to consider during this process and procedure. Southern California Reproductive Center articulated what patients may feel prior to the treatments:

"Many patients find themselves feeling a lot of anxiety around starting the IVF cycle... Taking new medications and experiencing new medical procedures is not easy, and the entire process of fertility treatment can seem invasive. Finally, the biggest stress for most patients is the fear that the cycle will fail. While fertility treatment can transform your chances of a successful pregnancy, it is an unfortunate fact that there are no guarantees. It is not uncommon for a woman to go through multiple attempts before getting pregnant, and with so much invested emotionally, physically, and financially the disappointment of an unsuccessful cycle can be crushing."

Many may feel intimidated by the journey that entails alternative fertilization, but there are also ways to help prepare for the process. One way is to continue a transparent dialog with your partner as well as your doctors. Ask for all information upfront to process with your partner prior to each step.

Additionally, a level of uncertainty about treatments and the desire to become pregnant can be a natural part of the journey. Acknowledging that fertility treatment is stressful allows a couple to ask for help and find healthy coping skills. Furthermore, Rachel Gurevich, Very Well Family, indicated:

"Research has found that feeling stressed about treatment does not ruin your chances for treatment success... They found that pre-treatment anxiety or depression did not affect pregnancy rates. The women with high anxiety were just as likely to conceive during treatment as those with lower anxiety."

Never ignore the presence of stress, anxiety, or depression; again, always continue a transparent dialogue with your doctor, and get the help needed throughout treatment, pregnancy, and after the birth of a child. Though the aspect of emotional stress brought about by these factors is present, it is not the only stressor that may arise; mental and financial stress could also play a role.

Financial Stress

Alternative conception comes with its own unique stressors, and to factor in the cost may overwhelm most—so much, it can deter couples from creating a family. One way to potentially reduce the stress is to try to understand the process. There are so many variables that go along with alternative conception that a couple may not know where to begin. Depending on each individual couple's needs and their own unique process, the quotes for cost vary. Where does one begin? Very

Well Family pointed out a few good questions to ask when getting a quote for IVF:

- Additional reproductive technologies you may need, like ICSI, PGT, assisted hatching, testicular sperm extraction, etc.
- Any pre-IVF fertility testing or consultations
- Cryopreservation of any extra embryos
- Fertility drugs
- Mock embryo transfer
- Pregnancy testing
- Ultrasound monitoring and bloodwork
- Yearly storage fee for those frozen embryos

As indicated above, there are many variables to consider, and if a couple has never been down this path, they won't know what needs to be asked or understood prior to deciding upon the journey.

Take note that all the above questions may vary if the alternative conception path is not IVF and is merely assistance in getting pregnant through other alternative means (e.g., solely medication, sperm retrieval, etc.). Again, there are countless avenues that couples may try in creating their family; the best suggestion is to be duly diligent and research the avenue chosen before embarking on the journey.

Now let us take a realistic glance at the cost for IVF and beginning a family. The following information can be intimidating, so it may be beneficial to take a deep breath while reading this data and be aware that everyone's process is different. The following information may not apply to everyone's journey, as some couples may need more help than others. CNY Fertility has outlined an overview of the basic costs:

- The cost of a basic IVF package: prices range greatly from as little as $4,700 at CNY to as much as $20,000, with the national average around $12,000. Note: national average may not include medication cost.

- The total cost of a single IVF cycle: At CNY total cost for IVF cycle is usually $8,000 but can go over $30,000 at some clinics, with a national average of around $20,000. Note: national average may not include medication.

- The total cost to bring home a baby with IVF: The cost to bring home a baby could be as low as one cycle, if that cycle is successful, though it is safer to plan for an average that accounts for two IVF retrievals and a few FETs. At CYN, the price range is between $16,000 and $20,000. The national average is in the range of $40,000 to $50,000. It is not uncommon to encounter those who have spent over $100,000 on treatment.

Readers may want to take a moment to absorb the intense information that has been revealed. This information was implemented for the sole purpose of giving a realistic view of costs, not to promote or endorse any facility. Always research all doctors, facilities, clinics, and other variables that will coincide with the journey; it is best for each couple to understand all aspects of their choices and decisions made.

Male Perspective

Often, the female's perspective and process will be the focus of discussion during alternative conception, leaving the male's outlook on the sidelines. However, witnessing, understanding, and embracing both perspectives of the experience is a more holistic and healthy option. It has become clear that men are often affected by infertility regardless of where the biological or medical issue may fall.

Esmee Hanna and Brendan Gough reported, "For 40% of couples who can't conceive, the problems lies with the man. But despite this, fertility remains something that is traditionally viewed as a 'woman's problem,' with male infertility rarely spoken about." Subsequently, it is understandable that men struggle with coming forth about their experiences, feelings, and/or concerns regarding the entire concept around the journey.

Furthermore, Hanna and Gough indicated that while conducting interviews, one man stated that, "It made me feel less than a man at the time knowing I may never father a child." Additionally, a second man shared that, "For a while, I thought less of myself as a person and as a man. I felt it was nature's way of telling me there is something wrong with me and that's why I am not able to have kids." It has become clear that both parties within the coupled unit are affected, and each must be able to communicate without the fear of judgment openly and transparently.

Moreover, when the infertility issue falls on the woman, it still affects her partner. For example, Dr. Jamie Long, reported that one husband disclosed, "How he was upset because he could not 'fix' the situation; claiming that men are 'fixers' by nature, so this disrupts the natural order." Whereas within the same posting, "Another highlighted the cost of infertility treatment and how inconvenient the schedule of treatment was for him; he is a 'planner' and treatments did not make plans further than two weeks out." Now keep in mind these two examples are not the spectrum of emotions that a man may experience, and every man is different.

In fact, there is an in-depth and heartfelt example on Dr. Jamie Long's website from one husband who stated, "Yes, I also felt terrible for not being able to fix the situation for my wife; treatments are expensive, and scheduling can be inconvenient. However, these points did not touch the depth of my experience; it wasn't that simple to me. It was much more emotional." For anyone who would like to read the full post, please visit drjamielong.com.

In a study titled "'I was with my wife the entire time.' Polish men's narrative of IVF treatment," ethnographer and anthropologist Maria Reimann discovered that:

"While men, just like their partners, undergo difficult and painful emotions rising from infertility and involuntary childlessness, they accept their role in the treatment as supportive and auxiliary. At the same time, men tend to suppress their own emotions and feelings of anxiety, depression, and loss because they believe they need to be strong in order to support their partners. Moreover, the notion of male fertility is closely connected to the notions of sexual intercourse and masculinity. Male infertility is associated with impotence, and therefore carries the stigma and shame of failed manhood."

The above excerpt is from a scholarly article that is an interesting read and recommended to anyone who may want a more in-depth look at a male's perspective.

Female Perspective

The female perspective is very versed, yet it is still important for the couple to discuss and understand. The journey for a woman can affect multiple aspects of her health, including physical, psychological, emotional, and possibly spiritual, depending on religious beliefs. Spiritual beliefs will not be covered here, so one may want to discuss this aspect with their partner and/or spiritual counsel.

The following are direct exemplifications on women who have experienced the journey from Carina Hsieh's article, "What IVF Really Feels Like, According to 12 Women Who Did It." The full article can be found in the November 2017 issue of *Cosmopolitan* online.

Katy, age 32, stated:

"IVF was one of the most physically draining experiences for my body. I always felt like a pin cushion trying to find a new spot to poke with the injections. They never tell you that you will actually run out of spaces to inject the needle. My body would throb and ache from the medicine. I would have to manage the different emotions like anxiety, sadness, and frustration from the additional hormones I was adding to my body all day. But I wouldn't change it for the world because it got me where I am today with two beautiful little ones."

Kelly, Age 43, expressed:

> "Physically it wasn't bad for me. Mentally it was a mind f*ck. It's like secretly running a road race of indeterminate length while going about your regular life and the finish line is holding your baby. Could be a 5K (my first IVF experience) or an ultra-marathon where you fall flat on your face, realize you still can't see the finish line and need to get up, stop crying, and keep running (my second IVF experience). And while you are going through all of this, there is always someone innocently asking when you're going to have a baby or some woman joke-complaining about how if her husband just looks at her she gets pregnant. It's hard."

Allison, age 41, indicated her experiences were as follows:

> "I don't think anything can prepare you for the emotional and physical feelings of IVF. On the emotional side, it felt like PMS times 100. I would go through a rollercoaster of emotions. From crying one minute to laughing the next. Physically, I literally felt pregnant, and I looked it too. The hormones and injections made my stomach bloat as if I were about 4 months pregnant. In fact, someone asked me when my due date was... that was fun! And the exhaustion. I had two younger children at home,

and I was working. It was the type of exhaustion that you feel like you have to lay down or you are going to die."

As illustrated above, each woman may experience the journey differently, showing that it is subjective in every way. Some women may have no indication or exacerbations of illness or discomfort from the medications, whereas others may be affected greatly. With the psychological and/or emotional aspects, some women may not feel anxiety or stress during the process, whereas others may have a great deal of fear, anxiety, stress, and with the addition of hormones, these feelings may be exacerbated greatly. Therefore, transparent communication between partners and all medical professionals throughout the entire process of IVF is vital. It is all about teamwork. Win Fertility has expressed why the physical and psychological aspects affect women in a more in-depth way:

Physically

One of the major physical challenges for women undergoing IVF is the effects of fertility drugs needed to stimulate the ovulation, help the eggs mature, prevent premature ovulation, and help the lining of the uterus prepare to receive the fertilized embryo(s). These are synthetic hormones which can make a woman experience the feelings of intense PMS. Mood swings, hot flashes, and temporary weight gain/bloating are common, as are headaches, breast tenderness, and nausea. Some medications must be injected in different areas depending on which drugs are prescribed, leading to feeling like a "pin cushion," as mentioned above.

Psychological

The first treatment cycle has been found to be the most stressful for patients, partly because it is a new medical procedure and one may not know what to expect even if a fertility specialist explains the treatment. Stress peaks during the waiting period after the embryos are transferred, while the woman waits to find out if she is pregnant or not. The uncertainty of the outcome is likely to add more stress. The cost of fertility treatment is another cause of worry for many people.

Again, alternative conception is not an easy process, which is why prior to embarking upon the journey, a couple may want to learn as much as possible. The more variables understood, communication, realistic goals, and fine-tuned plans, the less stressed a couple may become.

Male and Female Comparison

Infertility and the alternative conception process are obviously stressful for both males and females. In fact, one study conducted by Liying Ying, Lai Har Wu, and Alice Yuen Loke, "Gender differences in emotional reactions to In-Vitro Fertilization treatments," indicated:

"Although both men and women experienced psychological distress during the treatment, gender differences existed. Women had elevated anxiety and depression levels prior to the treatment, which became even higher on the day of oocyte retrieval, pre and post embryo transfer, and during the waiting period before the pregnancy test. Men of the infertility couples reported elevated depression scores before treatment, which usually increased during the time spent waiting for the outcome IVF treatment. Both men and women had lower scores on positive affect before the pregnancy test. A failed IVF cycle had long-term negative psychological consequences for both spouses."

The most reliable and productive way to understand is to connect openly with your partner. Each of you will embark on various emotions throughout your journey together, bringing us to the next step: wellness.

Wellness

As previously discussed, both individuals need to be supported during the infertility and alternative conception process. That said, the first wellness aspect will outline how to support the female partner, but there are many other forms of wellness modalities that will be outlined to help both males and females through the journey.

Try to remember the following points are merely a few general suggestions, and speaking openly with your partner will be beneficial to each individual woman and her needs. Win Fertility has outlined three ways in which the male partner may support the female:

- Do not deny your feelings or hers: Men tend to compartmentalize their feelings about fertility and only deal with them when the situation forces it, such as during testing or doctors' visits. Men should not expect a female partner to feel the same way they do or to be able to hide their emotions. Women need to realize that not expressing emotions does not mean your partner does not feel them.

- Communicate more clearly: Many people have trouble expressing what they want. They are hurt that their partner does not "just know" what they need. Both partners need to work at communicating better during the stresses of fertility treatment. An easy way is to ask for what you want, in a nonjudgmental way, or to offer something you think your partner might like.

"Would a hug feel good?" or "Do you want to talk?" can open a door to comfort.

- Remember to comfort: Both women and men like kindness. Small things can be comforting in stressful times, whether it is a little gift, something they like, or talking about fun times they have had. A thoughtful card, ordering dinner out, taking on extra chores around the house— small things can say a lot. A little kindness goes a long way.

The above suggestions may seem obvious, but many forget to be present and witness their partners. This brings the next technique to implement during the infertility and alternative conception journey.

Mindfulness Practice

Adopting this practice during infertility and IVF may help a great deal in reducing stress and promote communication. Andreia Trigo discussed how mindfulness during IVF can help with emotions and mental health during treatments. Trigo stated, "Mindfulness is a mental state achieved by focusing one's awareness of the present moment. In this state, we acknowledge and accept our own feelings and circumstances without any judgment." She also recommended the book *The Power of Now* by Eckhart Tole as a valuable read.

Some of the benefits of mindfulness practice researched by Daphne M. Davis, PhD, and Jeffery A. Hayes, PhD, were:

- Reduced rumination
- Stress reduction
- Boosted working memory
- Focus
- Less emotional reactivity
- More cognitive flexibility
- Relationship satisfaction

To read detailed information on each subject of this research, please visit the American Psychological Association's web page on mindfulness (apa.org/monitor/2012/07-08/ce-corner).

There are many books, apps, and information on the Internet regarding mindfulness practice that one may acquire. Another wellness technique could be journaling, whether keeping a gratitude journal or a daily ledger of one's thoughts and emotions to release them from the body. How can journaling help, you might ask?

Journaling Practice

Journaling can be a very cathartic way of releasing tension and expressing one's inner thoughts and emotions. Sometimes simply writing things out releases the ruminating inner workings of one's mind, which can help release stress. Starting a basic journal, sitting for a period of time each day or even once a week, may also help in organizing thoughts to better communicate with one's partner.

First Steps Infertility Clinic offers this explanation regarding journaling to their clients:

"The thought alone of becoming pregnant can bring about different feelings. What more if you have to go through infertility? This can bring about big and hard feelings... Some people refuse to keep a journal about their infertility journey, and that's understandable. Why would you ever consider it a journey when you want it to be resolved immediately, right? Here are some reasons why it's still advisable: The memories fade, journaling is therapeutic, and it becomes a part of history."

The above information is an attempt to recognize that infertility is not just biological and that mental and emotional aspects need to be addressed as well.

The known benefits of journaling, whether it be a general journal of thoughts and feelings and/or a gratitude journal are well documented. Courtney E. Ackerman indicated, "Overall, journaling/expressive writing has been found to boost your mood/affect; enhance the sense of well-being; reduce symptoms of depression before an important event; reduce intrusion and avoidance symptoms post-trauma; and improve working memory." To read more about these benefits and others that Ackerman discusses in her article, and to get a free pdf download of positive psychology exercises, look up her name in the reference list.

There are many different wellness avenues one may take while walking through the infertility and alternative conception process. Depending on the health of the individual, it may range from walking, swimming, hiking, and bicycling, to mediation, tai chi, gratitude, and journaling practices. The best recommendations would be from a doctor who knows all the variables of treatment, medications, family medical history, and patient's medical history.

Testimonials

Struggled Before Mindfulness (Male)

Many think that infertility does not affect the man in the relationship; they're wrong. Watching my wife struggle and feel the pressure she put on herself left me feeling helpless. I wanted to fix it but knew there was nothing I could do. We continued to try getting pregnant but nothing; so, we went to a doctor.

After discovering that there was a medical problem, we agreed to get help, but that did not change the dynamics or the reality; especially emotionally. My wife and I are close and can talk about anything. So, I sat her down and pointed out what I saw happening to her and between us. What we discovered was that she was feeling shame from not being able to conceive, and she felt I was pulling away from her because I was trying to give her space because I did not know how to fix the issue.

We talked with a friend who is also a counselor, who recommended journaling separately and mindfulness practices. The journaling allowed us to collect our thoughts before openly sharing, and the mindfulness helped us remember that we both have our own experience. Once we began setting a schedule to do both the journaling and mindfulness, followed by check-ins with each other, we both felt less stressed over the reality.

We did take the doctor's advice to get pregnant, but for me, interacting with the medical team and all procedures were uncomfortable at times. My wife was better at dealing with all of this, but together we helped each other and did not judge each other's experience.

Meditation (Female)

Once we decided to take the IVF route to conceive, I understood that it may be stressful especially since I would be doing all the shots on my own; not all men are okay with injecting their wife with a needle.

So, every morning I would listen to calming meditative music from YouTube for fifteen minutes, and at night I would do the same before bedtime. I would also perform deep breathing exercises, and sometimes I would add essential oils to the process (i.e., lavender, or vanilla oil).

The doctor's visits were enjoyable because the team was so supportive, but the shots at times seemed a bit cumbersome; and the lumps from the progesterone injections in the hip became uncomfortable after a while.

I had to do this practice many times because we did not get pregnant the first few times, and I also had a miscarriage, so it has not been an easy road. However, I feel the mediation routine and speaking with my husband as each cycle passed allowed me to remain calm and focused.

We are still trying to conceive and have not decided to try again or get a surrogate this time around. But I can say, for myself, time taken out for my self-care by sticking to a daily routine of meditation helped a lot.

Chapter 3

Introduction to Conception and IVF

What is conception? The medical definition is as follows:

From the Latin *conceptio, conceptionis* meaning conception, becoming pregnant. The union of the sperm and the ovum; the onset of pregnancy marked by the implantation of the blastocyst into the endometrium.

One may think conception is an easy thing to accomplish, but it is quite the contrary; many variables need to line up for the exact point of contact with hormones, sperm, and egg even when done naturally. The natural process will not be elaborated here, but alternative conception, specifically IVF, will be discussed step-by-step.

Conception Options

First, a couple needs to discuss all variables of their specific case with their doctor and decide on the best route to accomplish their aspired outcome. That said, some options to consider may include: partner's eggs or donor eggs, partner's sperm or donor sperm, carry personally or surrogate, and In Vitro Fertilization (IVF) or Intrauterine Insemination (IUI). Another option could be egg stimulation through medication and natural sperm delivery through sexual insertion with partner. The doctor can help to answer each of these questions, but it is beneficial for the couple to discuss these options prior to the process.

Alternative Conception and IVF Procedures

When thinking about alternative conception, most may think IVF. The conversation around IVF seems to be a common dialogue these days. As Penn Medicine described:

"When you think of common fertility treatments, In-Vitro Fertilization (IVF) probably appears near the top of your list. There's a reason for that. IVF has been around for decades and you most likely already know the basic idea behind IVF: uniting egg and sperm outside the body in a culture. But there is so much more to IVF that happens before and after that."

The phrase "so much more" refers to the multi-step process of medications, egg retrieval, and sperm donation from partner or donor, injecting sperm into uterus or directly into an ovum, egg hatching, and implantation of embryo and/or blastocyst. There are also specific genetic tests prior to implant available as well, to find out more about this, consult with a fertility doctor.

The jargon a couple will hear during their journey is "IVF cycle," meaning medication and calendar followed by each step toward implantation. IVF cycle usually begins with first or second day of the menstrual cycle, depending on doctor's protocol, with medications; some medications may be implemented prior to menstrual cycle depending on what is necessary per individual case. Again, each specific case may implement different protocols, medications, and procedures for each patient.

Medications

The medication process may include oral pills, injections, and/or vaginal suppositories. Loma Linda University indicates:

"Typically, a patient will start with an IVF cycle by taking birth control for several days, then injectable medication to stimulate ovaries and produce eggs, followed by a trigger shot and egg removal; this process allows the doctor to control the menstrual cycle during treatment."

At first, the medications and the calendar schedule may seem very intimidating, but trust that the process becomes clearer and smoother with each dose. If a partner helps administer the medication, it eases the process and allows both parents to be involved.

As for specifics regarding medications, Loma Linda University indicates that a typical IVF treatment will involve a mix of the following medications:

- *Hormone contraception (birth control pills)*: these pills help regulate the menstrual cycle and prepare the reproductive system for IVF.
- *Prenatal vitamins*: recommendations include taking these vitamins with at least 400mg of folic acid when attempting to conceive. Herbal supplements should be avoided.
- *Lupron*: this medication enables the body to produce a higher number of viable ova.
- *Antagon (Ganirelix)*: this medication helps prevent premature ovulation.
- *Follicle Stimulating Hormone (FSH)*: these injections increase the growth of follicles in the

ovaries. FSH is often prescribed as Gonal-F; Follistim; or Menopur.

- *Doxycycline*: this oral antibiotic is used to treat infection, such as reducing bacteria in sperm. It also reduces risk of infection following aspiration of the follicles at time of egg retrieval.
- *Novarel*: this is a synthetic human Chorionic Gonadotropin (hCG) injection used to stimulate ovulation.
- *Prednisone*: this steroid medication is used to treat patients with anti-sperm antibodies and repeated pregnancy loss.
- *Progesterone*: this endogenous steroid and progestogen sex hormone synchronizes preparation of the uterine lining with the treatment cycle to ensure the uterus is ready for embryo implantation.
- *Estrace* (estrogen): this medication is used to supply estrogen and comes in tablet form for oral use, or as a vaginal suppository.
- *Valium*: this medication is an anxiolytic (anti-anxiety) and sedative medication offered prior to embryo transfer.
- *Microdose Lupron*: this medication is often used to stimulate ovarian response before stimulating them.

To put it simply, the doctor intends to get control of the reproductive system and its process to control each step for potential success with the aid of these drugs.

Ovarian Stimulation

Each woman may experience something different depending on individual infertility issue and medications needed. However, the general steps for ovarian stimulation and follicle development are similar in most cases. Coastal Fertility Specialists outline the specifics:

- The process starts with ovarian suppression using hormone contraception (birth control pills) and/or Lupron.
- Once ovarian suppression is achieved, then starts the ovarian stimulation recombinant Follicle Stimulating Hormone (FSH)
- The stimulation is monitored through ultrasounds performed every 3 to 4 days along with blood hormone measurements, including estradiol and progesterone.
- Once most of the follicles (pockets of fluid which typically contain ova) are in the 16 to 20 mm size, ovulation is triggered with human chorionic gonadotropin (hCG). This is also known as a trigger shot.

- Retrieval of the ova is performed 35 to 38 hours later.

At first, the calendar, administration of medications, and time schedule may seem stressful, but it tends to go more smoothly than anticipated once the couple falls into a routine. That said, feelings of uncertainty are normal during this process. If one is unsure of a step, it is always recommended to check in with the medical coordinator and chosen emotional support counselor if the couple has one.

Ova Retrieval

The next step in the process is egg retrieval, which may feel intimidating as the woman must be put under anesthesia to retrieve the developed eggs. This procedure is usually done in an office, with a doctor and professional anesthesiologist, and takes approximately 15 to 20 minutes for most cases. Once the procedure is over, the recovery time is a 24-hour window of downtime for most women. CNY Fertility in Syracuse, New York detailed the process accordingly:

- Ova (egg) retrieval is a surgical procedure done to remove the ova from a woman's ovaries undergoing Egg Freezing or In Vitro Fertilization (IVF). Surgery is a big and scary word, but the procedure is done in a minimally invasive way, meaning it usually has no scars, no stitches, and a short recovery time.

- It takes place approximately 10 to 12 days after the start of hormone-based-stimulation medication taken to make ovaries develop numerous ova.

- The procedure generally lasts 10 to 15 minutes from the administration of anesthesia to completion of the egg and retrieval procedure.

- Egg retrieval procedure recovery is generally minimal due to the type of anesthesia (MAC) and the minimally invasive nature of the surgery.

- Risks for an egg retrieval procedure itself are relatively minimal due to the mild nature of the surgery compared to other medical procedures. Still, some risks include bleeding, infection, as well as damage to the bowels and/or bladder.

- Following the egg retrieval procedure, the eggs will be taken to an embryology lab where they will either be frozen, fertilized and developed for 3 to 7 days inside the lab, or, in rare cases, loaded into an INVOCELL device for fertilization and development.

Keep in mind that everyone's pre-existing and own medical journey will also be variables to discuss with your doctor regarding the risks of the aforementioned procedure. If needed, take a few minutes to walk away from the book at this point to integrate the information thus far.

The process of IVF can be overwhelming at times, and it is completely understandable to want a break; self-care is vital during this process. Next is combining the egg and sperm, fertilization, for implantation.

Egg and Sperm Fertilization

There are several ways in which a couple may introduce the sperm to the egg depending on the route the couple and doctor have set forth. Some options listed by Stanford Health Care are: In Vitro Fertilization (IVF); Intracytoplasmic sperm (ICSI); Gamete Intrafallopian Transfer (GIFT); Zygote Intrafallopian Transfer (ZIFT); Assisted Hatching; Blastocyst Transfer; and The Donor Oocyte (egg) program.

Again, depending on medical history and infertility issue, the aforementioned list may not apply. However, a brief description, given by Stanford Medical Center, is as follows:

- Retrieved ova (eggs): the ova are placed in a laboratory dish with the motile sperm, where fertilization takes place. The fertilized egg develops 3 to 5 days in a special culture medium in a controlled environment and are then transferred to the woman's uterus for potential implantation and embryo development.

- Intracytoplasmic sperm: this is an effective treatment for male infertility. Following egg retrieval, a single sperm is injected into each egg.

- Gamete Intrafallopian Transfer: like IVF, but with fertilization taking place inside the women's own body. Following retrieval, the eggs are mixed with sperm and transferred immediately into the fallopian tube via laparoscopy.

- Zygote Intrafallopian Transfer: another variation of IVF, involves transferring pre-embryos into the fallopian tubes just 24 hours after In Vitro Fertilization.

- Assisted Hatching: this involves laboratory manipulation of the embryo to create an opening in its outer covering (zona pellucid). This technique may increase the chance of the implantation, especially in reproductive older women.

- Blastocyst Transfer: as with IVF the eggs are retrieved, fertilized, and allowed to develop 2 to 3 days in cleavage medium. The embryos are then transferred to blastocyst medium for 2 additional days before being transferred to the women's uterus.

- The Donor Oocyte: this method offers hope for women with difficulty in egg production or whose eggs carry a genetic defect (egg donation).

This list is a brief overview; if one is interested in further information, it is recommended to discuss it with their doctor or do additional research.

At this point, there are two other questions a couple may want to think about: whether to freeze additional eggs and sperm retrieved and whether the couple would like genetic testing done on the embryo or blastocyst prior to implantation. The genetic testing offered is called Preimplantation Genetic Diagnosis (PGD) and can be discussed fully with a personal doctor. Next is the implantation day and then eagerly waiting the thirteen days for the pregnancy test results.

Embryo or Blastocyst Implantation

At this point, it is normal for the couple to be both excited and nervous. Depending on the clinic and doctor's process, the day of implantation can go two ways. Some doctors implement ultrasound to view the process while implanting the embryo or blastocyst, where others do not. It will depend on the procedure used by the doctor that will dictate if the implantation occurs with a full or empty bladder.

The timing of Embryo Transfer (ET) can differ and may depend on whether it is a fresh or frozen embryo or blastocyst transfer. Transferring an embryo or blastocyst with guided ultrasound has been depicted well by Christina Dias from Reproductive Medicine Association of Connecticut:

- Fresh embryo transfer process usually takes five days after retrieval.
- Frozen embryo transfers usually take place six days after starting progesterone.
- Embryo transfer will not require any anesthesia.
- Most transfers require a full bladder.
- After a series of verifications to ensure you receive the correct embryo, the embryo(s) will be carefully loaded into a catheter, and the catheter is inserted through the vagina and cervix, and into the uterus with the guidance of ultrasound imaging.
- Embryo transfer is virtually painless, with some cramping possible.
- The patient will be advised to rest for a few minutes after transfer, and then the patient can get up, empty their bladder, and go home.
- There are minor restrictions. The best news is that the patient does not have to be on bed rest.

Once the transfer is complete and the doctor has given all instructions, it is vital to trust the process. From here, the most intimidating part is waiting for the pregnancy test. The best advice is to exhale, do not research anything on the Internet, do not try any home tests, keep your mind healthy by writing in a journal, take it slow and easy, and trust the process. Also try to remember every woman's process is different. Not all women get spotting, or cramping, or any symptoms, but they can still be pregnant; trust the process and wait for the blood test.

Most blood tests, depending on the doctor's protocol, can be anywhere from nine to thirteen days after embryo transfer. If the pregnancy test has returned a negative pregnancy result, then it is on to the second cycle.

However, if it is a positive pregnancy test, the couple continues medications for a set number of weeks. The couple will remain with the fertility doctor until approximately nine or ten weeks, during which time ultrasounds and blood test may be taken to monitor the pregnancy before transferring to their OB/GYN.

Testimonial

My Journey

Part I: God Knows My Heart

As a child, I dreamed of having a great education, a great marriage, and a house full of kids running around. I thought I did everything I was supposed to do. I graduated college, completed graduate school with a master's degree, and felt I had started my marital life off on the right track.

I married a Nigerian man; a first son who is a lawyer. His family is from an esteemed group of educators and politicians that had helped form what is now known as Enugu State, Nigeria. As first son, he is the father of the family and his role surpasses his father in the sense that the adult first son inherits the role of being the father to his father, once he becomes a man. This is customary in African tradition and culture. The first son is the heir to all property and holds the highest position of power within the family, so he must continue to reproduce; specifically, a male child.

I never knew how much pressure it was to have kids until I married a first son. From the moment I said "I do," I was expected to be pregnant within the first few months of the marriage. Pressure came from his parents, his Klansmen, and the Igbo community.

I suffered multiple miscarriages and stillbirths and was required to go through a series of cultural activities geared around removing "demonic spirits" that the tribe felt was preventing me from having a successful pregnancy. My husband refused to participate in any of the ceremonies and called it nonsense. I felt it was also a stupid idea but knew if I rejected the idea it would be viewed as disrespectful to my in-laws.

According to my in-laws, I suffered from a "spiritual husband" who was secretly impregnating me without my knowledge and causing me to suffer pregnancy losses. In the eyes of the elders, it was imperative that I go through this exorcism to kill off my spiritual husband.

I was placed in isolation for 7 days in my father-in-law's compound and provided multiple prayers to read while I fasted. On the third evening of my isolation, my mother-in-law mobilized a group of four women and three men to stay with me for the remainder of the isolation period. I was bombarded with loud and aggressive prayer, called names, and forced to drink holy oil, which was also poured into my eyes, ears, and nose. A second set of activities included deworming and confession.

After the 7 days of isolation, I was informed by the head "Prayer Warrior" that I would not have any more problems having children. My mother-in-law celebrated throughout the compound and cooked Egusi and Pepper Soup, while visitors came to join in the celebration of my newfound solution to my pregnancy losses. I was skeptical, doubtful, and discouraged, because I wanted to believe that my problem was solved, but in my heart, I knew it was rubbish. I do, however, appreciate the efforts of my in-laws, as they were trying their best to help me within their limited scope of understanding.

Many would say, "Why would you subject yourself to things you did not feel comfortable doing?" My response to that is, "I was desperate for a child." My desperation led me to infertility specialists in San Francisco, London, India, and finally Africa. My life became obsessed with having a child. I felt so much pressure that I became severely depressed and had multiple hospitalizations for suicide attempts. I was convinced that if I did not have a child, I would die. I certainly felt my marriage would end, so I prepared myself for a life of solitude and isolation from the world.

Usually when a woman cannot produce a male child, the husband has the right to choose a second wife, and that reality loomed over my head. The thought of losing my husband because I didn't have a male son consumed my thoughts constantly and became my burden.

Prior to traveling abroad for infertility treatment, I was a patient at a Fertility Clinic in San Francisco, and after three unsuccessful treatments, I opted to get a surrogate. She was referred by my physician. She was a white woman, and ironically, we had the same name. She had a young son who had the same name as my husband, and they also shared the same birthday. I thought to myself, *This must definitely be the right person! It will finally happen for me!* I celebrated because I knew she is white, we have the same name, and her son's name and birthday are identical to my husband's. Somehow, I felt that her whiteness was assurance that things would work, but sadly it wasn't.

Her uterine lining was too thin, so she was

disqualified to be my surrogate. I tried again with another round of treatments, and multiple embryos were transferred inside of me. I did get pregnant, and I was immediately put on (sic) bed rest. I carried my son up until the six month and I delivered him dead.

His name was Tobechukwu; the English translation means "Praise the Lord." This tragedy did not make me Praise the Lord, not one bit. I was angry! I held him in my arms, yes, I held MY FIRST SON. To everyone else he was a dead fetus, but to me he was my son. I watched as his skin turned black right before my eyes. I took a photograph of his limp body, and I continued to hold him. I needed that picture as a final reminder of what he meant to me; what he represented. His short life was evidence to me that I was in fact a mother! I was a woman with the ability to reproduce. After all, we are put on this earth to procreate, but for me, it felt like it would never happen. *Why?* I wondered. What had I done that warranted me to continue to produce dead babies?

That was the question that circulated among my community; a question that was often asked through whispers and stares, body language, and avoidance when I encountered fellow wives at cultural events.

I stopped going out and became a recluse. I avoided watching television because I hated seeing Pampers, Huggies, and Toys R Us commercials. It crushed me to see pregnant women. I was not angered by them; I was just terribly sad. I felt useless. I made my bedroom my fortress, as well as my torture chamber. I would close myself off from people for weeks at a time. I refused to talk; I stopped bathing and combing my hair. I would pull out Tobechukwu's photograph, staring at him as I lay in the bed, mourning over my loss.

I stopped attending mass because I was angry with God. After all, God kept disappointing me. I saw no reason to fellowship. I was bitter, and I was in a deep pit. I had a funeral for my son at the Catholic cemetery in San Pablo. My mother-in-law didn't want the funeral because she felt that dead babies were evil spirits that should be forgotten. A mother in Igbo culture has a very specific relationship with her first son. He is not only her son, but also her husband, so she is actually considered the first wife and can make decisions to overrule the wife.

I wanted a funeral, and my desire to have one created resentment and was an act of defiance in the eyes of my in-laws, but I needed it for myself. When the service was completed and it was time to leave, I saw the groundskeeper putting my son's tiny little casket into the ground. I stayed and I waited to see the entire process, but I was encouraged to leave by family members. I refused to leave, and I sat and waited for the dirt to cover his grave.

My husband tried to be as supportive as he could, but he was torn between culture, ego, and confusion.

He could have taken the easy way out and just got a second wife, but he chose not to because it would have created bigger problems and because of the love he had for me.

The truth of the matter is, the marriage suffered, the relationship deteriorated, and our lives became a hidden battle that we no longer fought together.

After Tobechukwu's death, things really changed for me. I came to the resolve that I would never have male child. I learned to accept that my marriage was basically falling apart because I could not live up to my end of the deal. Family and friends would contact me from time to time and encourage me to do whatever I had to do to get a son. I never understood the relevance of that until an elderly man explained the meaning behind the statement.

The absence of not having a son in Igbo culture meant that I wasn't really a complete wife, meaning women could continue to pursue my husband, and also meaning he could continue his pursuit of finding a woman that could give him a son. His behavior changed and he began to treat me like I was a burden, and that the reason for the losses were somehow connected to a flaw within me.

Chapter 4

Transfer to OB/GYN

If you have successfully transferred from the fertility specialist to the OB/GYN, then congratulations are in order. If you have not, and you are not pregnant the first cycle, do not despair. It may take a few tries to accomplish the desired outcome.

If the couple's pregnancy test comes back negative, they could discuss a mock cycle to dial in the medications to be more confident that the uterus environment is receptive to the implant.

So, what now? As indicated by Fertility Associates of Memphis:

After the completion of the series of ultrasounds and blood tests through nine weeks or so of gestation, there is a high degree of confidence that a pregnancy is healthy and viable. At this time fertility specialists will often refer patients to their general OB/GYN for the remainder of their prenatal care and delivery.

OB/GYN

Once the couple transfers from the reproductive specialist to their general doctor, they will continue appointments approximately every four weeks, or more if needed. It is best to contact one's OB/GYN at about seven or eight weeks to make sure an appointment is lined up for the transition period at nine or ten weeks. Sometimes it is difficult to get an appointment right away, and it is best for the couple to call in advance for a smooth transition.

There are a few other aspects to think about when transferring. Jackie Gutmann gives an overview of things to keep in mind:

- You won't see your OB/GYN as often as you did your fertility specialist.
- You should get a copy of records and bloodwork, particularly since you may have already had much of the testing your OB needs.
- You should ask that your records be sent to you; that way, you will always have a copy.
- You should confirm your due date with your reproductive specialist.

Each of the aforementioned items is the responsible route, and to add to these items, remember to continue the transparent communication on all levels with the OB/GYN throughout the journey. This would also include all physical, emotional, mental, and spiritual concerns, if any, as well as pre-existing medical conditions.

From this point forward, the couple would progress as if it were a normal pregnancy journey and implement each exciting tradition that they wish to carry out. However, if the couple has chosen to use a surrogate to carry their baby or babies, then the process may be completely different.

Surrogate Birth

This process is a bit more arduous due to the multiple factors that are involved, but if this is the intended parents' route, most go with an agency to provide structured guidance. That said, some couples may go with a family member or friend as a gestational carrier. The details of this process are discussed more in the next chapter. The relationship, process, and procedures of the journey are outlined here.

There are many options for who the gestational carrier may be, and this should be discussed prior to signing contracts. If an agency is implemented to attain a surrogate, it is called the matching process. However, if the couple chooses a known carrier, then specifics and aspirations can be set forth prior to implantation. Note that even if the gestational carrier is someone the couple knows, it is always best to write every detail out in a contract and retain a lawyer who specializes in surrogacy law.

When using a gestational carrier, the intended parents must file specific paperwork with the hospital and county court system to ensure the baby is the sole responsibility of intended parents, and not the gestational carrier. Complicated, right?!

Some options that the intended parent may want to think about regarding participation during their journey:

- Implantation day
- Doctors' visits
- Delivery day
- Cutting the umbilical cord

Some agencies detail what the intended parents can be a part of, and with that information, the agency will help match a surrogate who may fit. However, there are other surrogates who are not comfortable with an open process, and that type of relationship may fit better for couples who want to be less hands-on.

An additional factor to consider is location; some surrogates may live in a different state or country. Each couple may want to sit down and discuss what may work best for them, and what their desired contact with the agency, surrogate, and baby process would look like.

When choosing a surrogate, it is always best to ask if she has been a prior surrogate. If yes, be sure to get all medical and medication cycle records sent to your fertility doctor. If you are using a first-time surrogate or a known carrier who has not done IVF, it may be wise to discuss doing a mock cycle first to dial in medications for the best chance of a positive outcome for implantation.

What is the first step to the process of surrogacy? The couple will first need to decide who will carry their child. If it is a friend or family member, there may not be a need for an agency. But again, it is always wise to get everything in writing—such as a contract by a lawyer who knows surrogate law. If a surrogate is used, then going through an agency will be required. Attaining a surrogate with an agency may be different depending on how each agency goes about their process. For example, *Find Surrogate Mother* indicated:

> During the process of choosing a Surrogate Mother, you should interact with the surrogate before making a decision. You will want to discourse your specific expectations and her individual needs and anticipations... If working with a clinic they will provide medical records for their presented Surrogate Mother. If you have precise preferences

concerning your surrogate, the clinic will try to meet these requests within reason.

Okay, now the surrogate or known carrier transfers to OB/GYN; if going with an agency, each surrogate usually gets a case manager, but at very least coordinates all doctor's appointments with agency. For example, as indicated by International Surrogacy Center:

> Surrogate released to Personal OB/GYN: It is your responsibility to inform the agency of OB/GYN to be treated for prenatal care. It is your responsibility to inform the agency of the OB/GYN information and the date and time of your first appointment... From this point, you will be the means of information between the OB doctor and intended parents. Agency requires the surrogate to keep us updated throughout the pregnancy with appointment dates and anything else that would be considered important information. Please make sure the OB doctor and hospital is in network of insurance.

Again, some agencies have a case manager who works directly and closely with the surrogate and is the go-between for intended parents. A big point here is to make sure that the doctor and hospital are covered within the health insurance network. Additionally, at about 26 weeks, the intended parents may request a 4-D ultrasound of their baby, but this will cost extra.

Furthermore, it is very important to make sure the paperwork "Judgment for Parental Rights" is filed by approximately 24 weeks; this must be done by the surrogate lawyer who wrote up the contract.

Now it is time for delivery, and the presence of the intended parents if they so choose. Prior to this date, the agency should have consulted with the OB/GYN and the hospital to make sure all the parties involved are aware that the delivery is a surrogate process.

At this point, some intended parents may decide to wait until after their baby is born to connect with the agency and greet their child, and some may want to be a participant at delivery. This is all a personal choice and need not be judged. Here is an example of being present during childbirth as stated by International Surrogacy Center:

Intended parents may wish to be present during childbirth. If the surrogate requires a cesarean, the doctor will usually allow only one support person present during the surgery. If a cesarean is required, the surrogate mother will inform us of who she prefers to be in the room with her. Normally this is not a problem to have the intended mother or father in the room, but in case of complications, the surrogate may want her own support person in the room with her for support.

There is so much to consider when choosing to have a surrogate or known gestational carrier. However, it is a blessing that another woman can or even would carry to help a couple create a family.

There are still many things to consider if choosing a gestational carrier or surrogate, because there are different laws, protocols, and procedures within each state and country. If a couple is to choose a carrier, it is wise to always get specialized legal advice in the state or country they are choosing to attain surrogacy. Be sure to retain an attorney who specializes in surrogacy law, and be sure he/she understands the laws in both your state/country and the state/country the surrogate or known carrier resides within. Due diligence is strongly suggested, as well as getting references and checking with the law board before retaining anyone.

Testimonials

Surrogate I

I became a surrogate for several reasons. I had just given birth to my second child. I got to the hospital and had him in less than 30 minutes later—1 push. I felt like I could climb Mt. Everest. The nurse said she'd never seen anything like that, and I should consider being a surrogate. I was taken back at the time; I literally just gave birth.

Fast forward about 2 years, and I had been thinking about that comment ever since. I decided to talk to my husband about it. He said he already knew I wanted to become a surrogate and was very supportive. I was also adopted from when I was a day old. My parents are my parents, and they are the best parents anyone could have. My mom was infertile, but they never figured out why and it was the 80s, so surrogacy wasn't a common thing back then. I have always been so grateful for my birth mom for giving me up. I have had the best life, and obviously she wasn't in a place to take care of me. Being a surrogate gave me a chance to give back to someone what I had been given a chance at a happy life.

I contacted a surrogate agency my friend had gone through. The agency owner came for a visit to my house to meet the whole family. She went over the process. It was several months before we were matched with a couple; the agency does a great job to match like people with the same ideals together. My husband and I then had to go get a psychological evaluation. That was a bit weird, because neither of us had been to a therapist before and didn't know what to expect. Needless to say, we passed and set up a meeting with the intended parents.

The meeting took place at a restaurant with my husband, the surrogate director, the case manager, intended parents, and myself. It was really weird at first—a bit like a blind date, I imagine. But we all clicked immediately. They were such wonderful people who suffered many miscarriages and, much like my mom, the doctors couldn't figure out why. We both agreed to move on with the process.

The next step was to go have a lot of bloodwork and a map of my uterus. Needles don't bother me in the slightest, and I've always given blood, so the bloodwork was a piece of cake. The mapping of my uterus was uncomfortable as they put a balloon and pumped it up to map it. All the tests came back just fine except for the cytomegalovirus (CMV) test. I was positive, which just meant I needed to wait until I was negative.

Several months later, I was still positive, which didn't make sense to me or my doctor. I asked my general practitioner (GP) if he could test me, because the medical facility where I had the tests at said I was still positive. My doctor asked for a specific test that would tell us if the CMV was active or I was immune. Turns out I was immune and the test the facility was using flagged for active or old infections.

Now was the time to do contracts. The contract was long and repetitive for good reason. I had my own lawyer who went over the whole thing with me. Contract was signed and notarized. In the middle of this, I was laid off from my job; the dentist I worked for was going bankrupt. Added stress, but I decided to continue with the process and look for a new position at the same time. Dates were set for the transfer and medications were sent.

I interviewed with several places for a job at a dental office and got offered several positions. I accepted a position with a dentist, and it was a woman my same age with little kids too. I decided I'd have to be upfront and let her know that I had a surrogate transfer scheduled in the next month. She was so supportive and thought it was wonderful. I knew that I would be happy and supported at my new job. I am still at the same position 4 years later, happy and very supported by the whole staff.

Medications started—a little needle in my stomach every morning for a few weeks. After that, a very large needle with viscous liquid was injected into my hips every day until I was 10 weeks pregnant.

The transfer was done with both intended parents and my husband in the room. We had decided on transferring 2 embryos: a boy and girl. The process was amazing, and we saw them wake the embryos up, suck them into the transfer tube, and get placed in my uterus. It made me realize how amazing it is that anyone gets pregnant; it seems like the stars have to align and everything has to go right.

We waited a few weeks to test to see if I was pregnant. I was. At that point I knew, because my body felt tired, and I was not really interested in eating (I love to eat!). Next, we did an ultrasound about a week after and saw the most amazing two little heart flickers. Both embryos had taken. The intended parents were cautiously excited, as they'd had so many losses. Thankfully, these two little babies stayed and grew. I was so happy for the parents. After knowing each other for a year at that point, they had become friends of ours.

The doctor visits were about the same as with my own children. After 10 weeks, I got to go to my normal OB, which was so nice because it was 5 minutes from my house instead of 1.5 hours away. The intended parents came to most of my appointments with the doctor, and the case manager came to all the appointments.

It was weird being pregnant and not preparing for a baby—so much less stress. I would get a lot of comments at the end of pregnancy about my cute belly; it really stuck out there with twins, but not too much more than my own kids. I always loved telling strangers that the babies weren't mine. Their confused faces led me to explain the situation and have a good conversation about surrogacy. I think I informed a lot of people about what it actually is and why people do it.

The pregnancy was pretty easy, just like with my own kids. I did have more pressure and my feet swelled a lot near the end. I am a runner, so I continued to run up until I gave birth just like I had done with my previous pregnancies. Near the end, I was having to go to the hospital every other day to have the babies checked. They thought one baby was bigger than the other (in reality, they weren't that much different).

I had my 37 weeks check with my doctor and the intended parents. I was about 3cm at that point, and I knew those babies were coming soon. I had never dilated with my own children before I went into labor; I'd just went from 0 to 10cm in about 7 hours with both. I joked to the parents that I'd see them later and went back to work. I told my boss and coworkers I thought the babies would come the next day. We all laughed, as I didn't seem like I was in labor.

Sure enough, about 7 p.m., I was pretty sure I was having contractions. I called the intended parents, case worker, and my mom. My kids were dropped off at my parent's house, and off to the hospital we went.

Here is my birth story: Friday I was 3cm and 37 weeks with twins. That night I went into labor, I was Group B Strep (GBS) positive so I had to get to the hospital ASAP to get the antibiotics. My husband and the parents all met at the hospital.

I was 4.5cm and admitted. Went to 7cm by 12 a.m. and stalled. Labor didn't hurt at all, so we all tried to sleep. After I walked the halls, etc., I started Pitocin in the morning about 10 a.m. The babies weren't stressed, but I was tired.

Things picked up slowly, and by 12:30 p.m., the contractions hurt a little. By 1 p.m. (Saturday 1/13), the contractions were consistent and painful. At 1:45, really painful. I should say my ideal birth plan was no pain meds and everyone in the room! Checked I was 7cm still.

After the nurse left, I was sure I had to push. I told everyone and they grabbed the nurse in the hall. She had to have measured wrong, because it was 20 seconds later, she checked, and said don't push.

The twins were born in the operating room (OR). There was a lot of running doctors and nurses. My husband and the parents had to throw their OR clothes on. They wheeled me to OR, and about 5 contractions later—me on my back w/o my husband to push on my hips for counter pressure.

Then, all 15 doctors and nurses as well as my husband and the parents were there. Three pushes later, a baby boy was out (it was an active 5 pushes, but they had me push without a contraction and it was hard or productive for those two).

They then threw the ultrasound on me and said don't push (again, a pretty bad feeling when you need to do so and can't). They found the girl and said, "Okay, push..." She flew out of me; I don't think I even pushed her.

Both babies came out healthy, and the look on the parents' faces was priceless! Baby boy was 5.5 lbs., and baby girl 5 lbs. 14 oz.

I am so happy everything went as planned. I told the nurses and doctors to be ready, but obviously they didn't believe me until it was a running situation; we had a great time in the hospital. I loved visiting with the babies and parents, and having my own room!

All in all, it was the most amazing experience of my life. The look on the intended parents' faces as they held their babies was one of such love. I pumped breast milk for the babies for the next year. Both babies were fed breast milk for their first year. The parents, my husband, and I remain friends. We keep in touch all the time, and it is fun to see those babies grow. They will be 3 in a few weeks. Because of COVID, we aren't able to visit every few months, but we keep in contact by texting and sending pictures.

My journey is complete! Such a perfect and wonderful experience!

I am currently in the process of my second journey with a different couple. I can't wait for them to meet their baby. I feel so blessed that I am able to safely carry children and have relatively easy labors and deliveries.

Surrogate II

When it came to this surrogate, she felt it would be easier for her to answer specific questions rather than write out a testimony. So, the following is how she chose to contribute to help others.

What prompted you to look into being a surrogate?

Being a surrogate is something I had always wanted to do. I can't pinpoint the exact time of what made me want to become a surrogate... I knew from when I was a teenager, and my 13-year-old cousin had gotten pregnant, that I wanted to be able to provide a family for someone other than myself... I know I had seen a Lifetime movie at some point in high school that directed me in understanding what surrogacy was. By this point, that same cousin had another child by another man, and all I could think was there are deserving people out there struggling to have a family, yet here is my young cousin having babies irresponsibly... It just made me so frustrated!

When did you first think about becoming a surrogate?

I later learned that surrogacy did require you to have had a child of your own first. I had my son in 2009 and was married at the time. My then-husband had a previous child with his previous wife, and long story short, his daughter had only lived for a few hours. Needless to say, he did not fancy the idea of me wanting to be a surrogate, which was understandable with his history of loss. Once we divorced, becoming a surrogate was one of the very first things I decided to look into! I was 25 years old at that time and had decided to pursue surrogacy because I knew it was something I wanted to do.

Why did you want to carry another woman's child?

Between watching family members who had children that I didn't think should have and knowing deserving people were out there unable to have children of their own in the traditional way, I knew I could help. Why wouldn't I? Giving the gift of life and helping to create a family is the most fulfilling thing I have ever done with my life!

How was the process for you?

I had decided to go through a surrogacy agency and found an amazing one to do my surrogacy journeys through! The process is different with every surrogacy. This specific agency has a matching process that I greatly appreciate, as it makes sure to try and let the journey be enjoyed as much as possible between the intended parents and the surrogate! I was always very open and wanted all my surrogacies to be treated as though the intended parents were participating as much as possible. I always welcomed them at doctor appointments, encouraged them to feel any belly movements they were there for, and invited them into the delivery room to be a part of that as well!

How many times have you been a surrogate?

I have been a surrogate a total of 3 times.

How did the surrogacy journey(s) go?

I have been a surrogate a total of 3 times; each time was so vastly different as far as the experiences went. My first surrogacy, I ended up having twins! The pregnancy itself was perfect and uneventful. I can't say the process was the same, and I definitely learned a lot from it. After having the twins, I didn't hear much from the family until about 5 years later... The twins are doing great thankfully, and I was so happy to hear about them (and see pictures!).

My second surrogacy was absolutely the opposite! I have an amazing relationship with the parents, but it was a very rough pregnancy. I won't leave you in suspense; everyone is happy and healthy! During that surrogacy, we had learned about a blood issue. But thankfully, with a lot of monitoring, the baby did amazing!

My third surrogacy was a mix. I don't hear much from the family, which is always a little sad. The pregnancy was uneventful, which is always a great thing!

How was it to interact with the intended parents?

Each interaction is so different with each family. My first journey was met with a lot of disappointment and constant excuses/cancellations as to why they were unable to make appointments. It was very sad to me, and it did not give me the feelings I was looking for in a surrogacy journey. This was an easy pregnancy, but a rough interaction with the intended parents as I was not feeling heard (i.e., I would explain that sweets made me nauseous, but when they would show up for appointments, they would always bring chocolates or baked goods).

My second surrogacy, the parents were just amazing! They encouraged us hanging out and included my son in these interactions. I felt like they really wanted to get to know me, and that I wasn't just a "human incubator." I cannot express enough gratitude for this family.

My third surrogacy was rough for multiple reasons—the biggest being at 37 weeks of pregnancy, my house burnt down in the Tubbs Fire, and we were told to evacuate at 1:30 a.m. We had 20 minutes to wake up, find things in the dark, and drive away from our home as fast as we safely could. The surrogacy up to that point was uneventful, but it's hard to explain to anyone how you're feeling when your entire life gets tossed upside-down, and the intended parents didn't understand why I was struggling at the end of that surrogacy.

Was it difficult to give the baby to the intended parents?

It was not difficult at all to hand over the baby to the intended parents. I can't even begin to explain the joy I feel when this happens. The look on the new parents' faces, and the undeniable joy I can see emitting from the new family—it's just a feeling I can't describe. An utter sense of joy and accomplishment. To know I was a part of that process, to be able to bring such joy to a family. I really can't begin to try and put into words how it feels to give that to someone.

What is the process to be a surrogate, and what do both parties do? (i.e., is everyone at doctor's appointments, the hospital, etc.)

The process to become a surrogate includes multiple doctor appointments and a psych evaluation, which is not just for the surrogate but the intended parents as well. Once everyone is given the go-ahead after the psych evaluation, the surrogate generally goes to the IVF doctor, and basically makes sure her uterus is in good standing for a pregnancy—as well as lab tests to make sure everything looks good.

If there is a green light, generally the surrogate starts medications to basically trick her body into thinking she is already about 3 months pregnant at the time of the "transfer" (when the IVF Doctor implants the embryo). The surrogate stays on these medications for a couple months until the doctor feels it is safe for her to stop them, and her body automatically takes over making the appropriate hormones to sustain the pregnancy.

At this point, generally the surrogate moves on from the IVF doctor to an OB/GYN—almost like a graduation! The intended parents and the surrogate generally discuss at the beginning (before transfer of the embryo) what kind of relationship they would like to move forward. I always loved the idea of having the intended parents being at as many doctor appointments as possible, and to enjoy the pregnancy as much as they can during the entire process, which includes the delivery. It's quite an experience, and I would hate for them to miss out on that.

What did you get from being a surrogate? (i.e., emotionally, mentally, spiritually)

I can't begin to describe the feelings or emotions I get from being a surrogate. I understand it is seen as a huge selfless act, and I acknowledge that 100%. But the joy and elation I get from being able to provide someone with a child of their own, to create or expand a family— the feelings are just indescribable. I really wish I could continue to be a surrogate several times over!

Chapter 5

IVF Cost

Costs were briefly discussed in a previous chapter. However, this chapter will outline the potential cost in more detail. Remember that everyone's journey will be unique, and the financial scope will be on a spectrum depending on what is needed for individual couples. The range of cost for infertility to delivery lands on a huge spectrum—anywhere from $12,000 to $140,000 dollars depending on clinic cost, number of cycles, procedures, medications, ultrasounds, and donor and/ or surrogate, and even what state, or country in which the process is implemented.

CNY Fertility has broken down the average IVF cost in detail:

- Base Cost: $12,000
- Medications: $4,000
- ICSI: $1,500 (for some couples)
- Assisted Hatching $500 (for some couples)
- Cryopreservation and Storage $600 (for some couples)
- Frozen Embryo Transfer: $4,000
- Genetic Testing $4,500 (for some couples)
- Totaling: $20,000

CNY Fertility also stated, "When talking about the average cost of IVF: what it cost to actually bring home a baby. That number depends largely on the cost of a single cycle, but some studies report averages of $50 [to] 60,000."

Note that this is for one cycle, and it is not uncommon for the first cycle to fail. Infertility and IVF, or any alternative conception, can be complicated and may take many tries before a success; and that is still not guaranteed. Additionally, the aforementioned information is a general overview, and each individual couple will face their own unique process that may present different financial variables.

A few things that may not be included in the clinics cost break down may include medications, pregnancy test, mock cycle, and ultrasounds. Again, depending on each individual's case, the cost for a cycle lands on a spectrum.

Medication

If the cost of medication is not included in the clinic's process, it may range upon a very wide spectrum depending on the couple's process. If the couple's desire is to try and conceive through intercourse and boost the female's egg count, that would cost less than proceeding with an IVF cycle. Again, everything depends on the individual issues that each couple is facing with their infertility journey.

As indicated by Extend Fertility, "The oral medication used in conjunction with timed intercourse or intrauterine insemination (IUI) are much less than the injectable medications for IVF; both medications are typically under $100 per cycle. However, the average fertility medication cost for IVF, egg, and embryo freezing cycles are $2,000 to $5,000."

It is also best to note that with some clinics, the pregnancy test following implantation is an additional cost from original quote. Additionally, other blood tests and ultrasounds, such as the blood test during second trimester known as Quad Marker Screening, that may be needed during the process with the fertility doctor may not be covered. It is always best to inquire about any further tests, procedures, and/or processes that may be needed for each case.

Agency and Surrogacy Cost

As if infertility and alternative conception was not stressful enough, now factoring in the potential of an agency and surrogate may induce unimaginable angst. Again, exhale. These feelings are normal. The best way to combat the anxiety that may occur is to attain all variables to make an informed decision.

Total Average Cost

Obviously, this may vary depending on each circumstance, agency, and process, especially if any additional factors are involved such as donor egg and/or sperm. That said, as stated by The Sensible Surrogacy Guide, "The average cost of surrogacy ranges from $120,000 to $150,000 in the United States, but low-cost options start at less than $100,000. Overseas surrogacy cost as little as $50,000 in Eastern Europe or South America, to $80,000 in Western countries like the UK, Greece, or Canada."

However, remember to research every aspect, especially when going to another country. Due diligence is key and investigating what is needed legally within each country and one's own state or country is vital to a smooth process. The Sensible Surrogacy Guide has outlined the process in-depth and seems to incorporate averages for each step and stage of the surrogate journey.

The surrogacy route can pose many variables, and most will be outlined below with an overview. However, remember that this is not an in-depth account—just some aspects to think about. The following aspects will include: agency fee, surrogate fee, legal fee, life insurance fee, screening fee, surrogate group fee, and potential fee information for insurance. Note that the insurance aspect can be complicated and may include additional fees over and above required payments, such as a percentage charged for using a surrogate.

Agency

Due to the complexity and multiple working parts of the surrogacy journey, most couples may choose to go through a surrogate specialist and agency. The agency will charge a fee and may vary depending upon state and logistical processes. An average cost solely for the help from an agency may run anywhere between $13,000 to $25,000, and it may involve additional costs if the agency is more hands-on or unforeseen issues arise with the pregnancy journey.

For example, as suggested by Cost Helper Health, the agency fee may be broken down as follows:

The International Assisted Reproductive Center in

Maple Grove, Minnesota, which estimates a total cost of $60,000, charges administration fees of $16,000—payable in an initial installment of $8,000 and two more of $4,000—with the rest of the expenses varying on a case-by-case basis.

It is worth mentioning that the initial fee is usually required upon registering to find and match with a surrogate, and in most cases is not refundable regardless of if pregnancy occurs or not.

Therefore, before going any further, note that the potential off the top—without considering any additional costs—may range from $13,000 to $25,000. The fee does not calculate the surrogate base fee, screening and psychological, health and life insurance, lawyer and filing fees for parentage, and any other unforeseen or additional costs such as childcare if the surrogate needs it or loss of wages if the surrogate is ordered for bed rest during the process.

Surrogate

Surrogate fees vary drastically depending upon multiple variables, such as: what state or country they reside in, if she has been a surrogate before or if it's her first time, if she will be carrying singleton or multiples, and so much more. For example: if she is a first-time surrogate carrying a singleton, her fee may range from $35,000 to $50,000 depending upon which state she resides in, and this can go up if she is carrying multiples. Note that this amount is merely her base fee and does not include everything else to attain a surrogate.

The Storks Nest Surrogate Agency, out of Indianapolis, outlined information on the average costs for a first-time surrogate:

- Gestational surrogate base compensation: $35,000
- IVF transfer and bed rest, etc.: $1,000
- Maternity clothing allowance: $750
- Monthly allowance in lieu of itemized cost (mileage, parking, vitamins, etc.): $3,000

The above itemized list does not include potential additional reimbursement costs such as childcare, loss of wages, loss of organ, Ectopic pregnancy, fetal reduction, etc. (for an in-depth look, follow the link provided in the reference list, or do in-depth research on this topic for your own state.) Remember that each state may charge depending on where the intended parents live.

Legal

There are many aspects the legal cost may cover, such as contract drafting and reviewing for both the intended parents and surrogate. Here, the intended parents will pay for their lawyer fee and a separate lawyer for the surrogate to review the contract. In addition, the lawyer will charge for establishment of parentage, which needs to be notarized and filed with the county. If the intended parents choose, the lawyer can also take care of the trust account needed for the entire process, for a fee, or the intended parents may choose a third party such as seed escrow account services. West Coast Surrogacy has organized some average costs for these items:

- Drafting of gestational surrogacy contract for intended parents: $2,000 to $2,750
- Review of gestational surrogacy contract on behalf of surrogate: $1,000
- Established parentage: $4,000 to $7,000
- Trust account management: $1,000

In addition to these fees, the intended parents must get a life insurance policy out on the surrogate. It is always wise to make sure this is noted and accounted for within the contract. It is also up to the intended parents to inquire about a nondisclosure agreement to be added to the contract if the couple does not want anyone knowing about the surrogacy transaction.

Screening and Psychological Support

The screening process will be conducted on everyone involved, including the surrogate's spouse or significant other. Psychological support is offered to the surrogate during the process of the pregnancy and surrogate journey. Furthermore, a medical screening will be done on the surrogate and their partner as well, but this will be done by the fertility doctor; if the couple wants more information regarding this aspect, they can inquire with their agency and/or fertility clinic.

West Coast Surrogacy has outlined some of the cost for the screening process as well as psychological support:

- Psychological Screening – surrogate, spouse, and intended parents: $1,000
- Criminal Background Investigation – surrogate and spouse: $126 to $402
- Medical Screening of Surrogate and Spouse – as determined by IVF physician
- Psychological Support – monthly surrogate support group, email, phone call: $2,500

These variables are in addition to the base fee for the surrogate and fees outlined above thus far.

Health Insurance

This section may induce some anxiety, so take as much time as you need to read and re-read. The insurance aspect is very complicated when having a gestational carrier. In addition, now that surrogacy has become more popular, the insurance companies can charge a percentage of the fee that is paid to the surrogate. For example, if the surrogate is in California and gets the base pay for being a first-time carrier at $50,000, the insurance company may charge a percentage toward that fee on top of all the regular costs to obtain insurance (i.e., monthly fee, deductible, and co-pays). Furthermore, the newborn may not be covered on the surrogate insurance agreement.

If an intended parent uses a specialized surrogate health care plan because their health insurance does not offer coverage for surrogates, they need to understand that the newborn is not covered. As indicated by IVF Conceptions, "Intended parents need to know that surrogate health insurance pays for surrogate pregnancy care and birthing but for newborn separate insurance is needed."

There are not many specialized surrogate health insurance providers, and many health care providers may not agree to surrogacy coverage. It may be best to line up the health insurance a couple would like to use prior to engaging with the surrogate route; this is the couple's choice. IVF Conception further stated, "There are around 5% surrogate health care plans that openly accept surrogacy pregnancy. Around 30% of insurance plans do explicitly mention that they do not cover surrogate pregnancy." Inquire about insurance and find out where your insurance company stands on surrogacy.

Surrogacy insurance can be a very worrisome aspect of the journey, and it is always best to speak with an insurance broker and get in writing what the insurance company will cover. American Surrogacy indicated, "Insurance companies have caught on to the growing trend of surrogacy—and have started writing policies that only cover a pregnancy within the family, not a surrogacy pregnancy. This is where it is key that a surrogacy professional completes an insurance review and gets an interpretation of the policy in writing."

In addition, keep in mind that surrogacy insurance can be costly. Some choices for surrogacy insurance may be Risk Financial or New Life. A general overview given by American Surrogacy outlined the following:

- Premiums can be approximately: $10,000
- For a single-child pregnancy, deductible can start at: $15,000

It is always best to inquire directly and share all variables the intended parents foresee taking (i.e., single or multiples, state or country residing, etc.). Also, it is strongly suggested to get everything in writing and attain a copy of the contract. Another very important variable to note is to make sure the doctor and hospital the intended parents want will be covered within the policy.

If the above two insurances are not a route the intended parent would like to go, Lloyds of London Surrogacy Insurance is an additional option. As indicated by Conceivable Abilities, "Lloyds coverage allows the surrogate to see any doctor that is mutually agreed upon by intended parents and surrogate, and the option to switch to a specialist if they prefer. Remember surrogate's own plan (Riskiest), individual plan (Unknown), and Comprehensive Surrogacy Plan (No Risk)." Again, it is suggested to get everything in writing and be sure a professional helps assist the intended parent, so no hidden costs arise due to inexperience and not knowing what questions to ask.

Life Insurance

It is required to obtain a life insurance policy on the surrogacy in case unforeseen issues occur during the pregnancy. As stated by Conceivable Abilities, "Although it may not be the most pleasant thing to think about, it is true that pregnancy is not without risk... This is in part why most reputable surrogate agencies require surrogates to obtain a life insurance policy. Our surrogates are required to obtain a policy within thirty days of their becoming pregnant. The policy must be for at least $250,000 (unless otherwise specified in the parties' legal agreement). Surrogates are, of course, reimbursed for this expense."

Intended parents are responsible for the life insurance policy cost and potentially other unforeseen costs along the surrogacy route. Always inquire if there are any further potential costs over and above those outlined in the original agreements. A few options may be Sagicor, Gerber, NY Life, or just asking your current insurance broker.

Okay, exhale. Take a moment to breathe, because it is very understandable to feel overwhelmed by all this information. If possible, try not to get into your head and ruminate. Asking why it may be so difficult for some and so simple for others will not improve the process; it will only create stress. Though it is natural to ask these questions, remaining on the path toward manifesting one's aspiration is best.

But if, after reading and integrating all the information, alternative conception is no longer the desired outcome, that too is okay. No judgment for either choice should be projected or made.

Testimonials

My Journey

Part II: God Knows My Heart

I decided to move back to Africa and pursue a surrogate. I reconnected with a former IVF physician because I knew the IVF treatments would be less expensive, and he was familiar with my history. We decided to use my eggs that were previously frozen. We also determined that the surrogate would live in housing which was located on the campus of the hospital so she could be supervised and monitored under the physician's care.

The surrogate was a stout African woman who had a young son. My husband and I paid her monthly medical costs and accommodations and gave her a monthly salary. Genetic testing was conducted, and everything appeared fine, yet I was skeptical and very suspicious of this woman. I had never met her, and she was someone arranged by my husband and the physician.

For a while, I wondered if she was my husband's mistress. It is not uncommon for men to have mistresses in African culture, so this question was not out of the ordinary realm of thinking, but I dared not ask.

Things seem to be going okay and the baby was growing and thriving, and I continued to monitor the progress of the surrogate. Part of the reason I had to remain a mystery is because had she known I was from America, she would have demanded more money for her services. I did not want to run the risk of her breaching the contract, so I never met her until the day of my son's birth.

Ironically, our first phone conversation was an uncomfortable discussion regarding her sudden change

of plans regarding her undergoing a C-Section. The
surrogate had decided one week prior to the scheduled
C-Section that she was not having a C-Section because
she felt uncomfortable with the risks of mortality. I
understood her concerns but had to remind her that
when she originally signed the contract, she agreed to
a C-Section birth. Now that she wanted to change it, I
was not happy. We exchanged words over the phone,
but there were no rude remarks and, at the end of the
conversation, we had all agreed to continue with the
original plan for the C-Section delivery.

On the day of the scheduled C-Section, the surrogate
disappeared. Let me say that again. She freaking
disappeared! She had left her housing unit and was not
answering any calls for a day and a half. I was frantic.
Where was she? Where was my baby? *WTF!!!!!*

I couldn't contain myself, so I immediately came to
the hospital and waited to see the physician to find out
more about what was going on with my baby. I waited
all night and the following next day.

Toward the evening, the surrogate showed up with a
baby wrapped in a dirty blanket. I noticed his features,
and there was no doubt that he was my son. My baby
had indentations around his neck from the umbilical
cord. It was determined that my son had sepsis. I was
furious, and I asked the surrogate where she had been
with my baby. She stated that she was at church all
night, and that the baby was born in the church and

that the members delivered him vaginally. I asked her who was the presiding physician and she said there was no physician available. I asked her what day was he born, was it yesterday or today? She could not answer. I almost beat her, but my husband told me to calm down. My son needed two blood transfusions and was on a serious antibiotic cocktail for the first three weeks of his birth. My son was born into suffering, but I thank God he is alive.

He was born in a church, which means he was surrounded by Christ, and for that I am grateful. In my life, I have been fortunate to see three miracles from Our Lord Jesus Christ. Chimobi is my testimony of the reward and miraculous love and mercy that God has for his children. He rewards us, even when we least expect it, and the reward is greater than we could have ever dreamed. For anyone struggling with pregnancy loss, please do not give up. There are many options and resources. The ingredients that have helped me overcome my depression, loss, and grief have been: Patience, Prayer, Tolerance, and Understanding (keeping one eye closed so you can learn to forgive yourself and others).

The English translation for Chimobi means "God knows My Heart"—and I thank God for knowing what I needed and knowing my heart.

Afurumgi Nanya Obim: "I Love You, Baby!"

About the Author

Mimi's first published work was her dissertation: *Bright Lights, Dark Shadows: An Integrative Literature Review of the Psychological Consequences of Celebrity and Fame for Entertainers*, which is currently being proposed for a documentary.

Her second published work was *Bright Lights, Dark Shadows: The Shadow of Celebrity and Fame.*

Her third published work was *Emasculated: Men Are Abused Too.*

Her fourth published work was *Death: Before & After, A Survivor's Guide.*

Her fifth published work was *Lurking in the Dark, Reality of the Times.*

Mimi lives in Sonoma County, California. She is an Advocate, Author, Speaker, and Consultant. She has been educated in multiple areas such as: Business, Clinical Psychology, Human Resources, and Computer Science. Her aspiration in life is to advocate for those who are not seen and encourage everyone to be their healthy self and participate in their own wellness:

Mind, Body, Heart, Spirit, and Sensuality. Currently, Mimi's journey has shifted and led her to empower individuals and couples along their journey of infertility to conception through alternative resources.

She may be followed at her website: mimipsy-d.com.

Other Books by Mimi Amaral

Bright Lights, Dark Shadows: An Integrative Literature Review of the Shadow Side of The Psychological Consequences of Celebrity and Fame for Entertainers, 2016, Published by ProQuest LLC

Bright Lights, Dark Shadows: The Shadow Side of Celebrity and Fame, 2018, Published by Crescendo Publishing LLC

Emasculated: Men Are Abused Too, 2018, Published by Crescendo Publishing LLC

Death: Before & After, A Survivor's Guide, 2019, Published by Crescendo Publishing LLC

Lurking in the Dark, Reality of the Times, 2020, Published by Crescendo Publishing LLC

Connect with the Author

Website
mimipsy-d.com

Email
mimi.psyd@gmail.com

Social Media
LinkedIn: https://www.linkedin.com/in/mimi-ama-
           ral-71696229/

Acknowledgements

First, acknowledgment and gratitude to Cosmic Alignment and Divine Guidance (AKA: Source/God). Without this divine guidance, none of this would have manifested.

"Always give credit where credit is due. Never allow someone else to take the gratitude, especially when they did not help manifest and only created chaos or made things harder."

~ Mimi Amaral

With Special Gratitude

To all volunteers for testimonies: So much gratitude for sharing your personal experiences to help others understand they are not alone.

To Dr. T. Owens-Gager: For your encouragement and editing all the books.

References

Ackerman, C.E. (2020). *83 Benefits of Journaling for Depression, Anxiety, and stress*. Retrieved from: www.positivepsychology.com/benefits-of-journaling/

American Pregnancy Association. (2020). *Signs of Miscarriage*. Retrieved from: www.americanpregnancy.org/healthy-pregnancy/pregnancy-complications/signs-of-miscarriage-916#:~:text=Miscarriage%20is%20the%20most%20common%20type%20of%20pregnancy,pregnancies%20may%20account%20for%2050-75%25%20of%20all%20miscarriages

American Surrogacy. (2020). *Intended parents where can i find surrogacy insurance*. Retrieved from: www.surrogate.com/intended-parents/surrogacy-laws-and-legal-information/where-can-i-find-surrogacy-insurance/#:~:text=Surrogacy%20insurance%20coverage%20is%20a%20complicated%20subject.%20Before,become%20more%20popular-%2C%20the%20rules%20began%20to%20change

Center for Disease Control and Prevention (CDC). (2019). *Infertility frequently asked questions: Is infertility common.* Retrieved from: www.cdc.gov/reproductivehealth/infertility/index.htm

Cleveland Clinic. (2016). *Infertility causes.* Retrieved from: www.my.clevelandclinic.org/health/diseases/16083-infertility-causes#:~:text=Infertility%20may%20be%20caused%20by,to%20certain%20chemicals%20and%20toxins

CNY Fertility. (2020). *IVF cost: Analyzing the true cost of in-vitro fertilization.* Retrieved from: www.cnyfertility.com/ivf-cost/

CNY Fertility. (2020). *IVF egg retrieval: Process, procedure, recovery, risks, and more.* Retrieved from: www.cnyfertility.com/ivf-egg-retrieval/

Coastal Fertility Specialist. (2020). *IVF Process Step-by-Step: Ovarian Stimulation.* Retrieved from: www.coastalfertilityspecialists.com/treatment/in-vitro/in-vitro-virtual-tour-step-2/

Conceivable Abilities. (2017). *Surrogacy health insurance: What you need to know.* Retrieved from: www.conceiveabilities.com/about/blog/surrogacy-health-insurance-what-you-need-to-know#:~:text=The%20Lloyds%20coverage%20 allows%20the%20surrogate%20to%20 see,plan%20%28Unknown%29%2C%20and%20 Comprehensive%20Surrogacy%20Insurance%20 %28No%20Risk%29

Conceivable Abilities. (2017). *Choosing surrogate life insurance.* Retrieved from: www.conceiveabilities.com/about/ blog/choosing-surrogate-life- insurance#:~:text=This%20is%20 in%20part%20why%20most%20 reputable%20surrogacy,%28unless%20 otherwise%20specified%20in%20the%20 parties%E2%80%99%20legal%20agreement%29

Cost Helper Health. (2020). *Surrogacy cost: How much does surrogacy cost.* Retrieved from: www.health.costhelper.com/surrogate-mother. html

Davis, D. & Hayes, J. (2012) *What are the benefits of mindfulness.* Retrieved from: www.apa.org/monitor/2012/07-08/ce-corner

Dias, C. (2020). *What to expect at your IVF embryo transfer a nurse's perspective.* Retrieved from: www.rmact.com/fertility-blog/what-to-expect- ivf-embryo-transfer

Extended Fertility. (2020). *Fertility medication costs (and how to lower them).* Retrieved from: www.extendfertility.com/fertility-medication-costs-and-how-to-lower-them/#:~:text=We%20advise%20our%20patients%20that%20the%20average%20fertility,doses%20of%20medication-%E2%80%94which%20means%20higher%20fertility%20medication%20costs

Fertility Associates of Memphis. (2020). *Transferring from fertility specialist to OB/GYN.* Retrieved from: www.fertilitymemphis.com/im-finally-pregnant-happens-next/

Find Surrogate Mother. (2020). *How do I choose a surrogate mother?* Retrieved from: www.findsurrogatemother.com/surrogacy/guide-for-intended-parents/how-do-i-choose-a-surrogate-mother

First Steps Fertility Clinic. (2016). *Going through infertility: How journaling helps.* Retrieved from: www.firststepsfertilityclinic.com/going-through-infertility-how-journaling-helps/

Grunebaum. A. (2020). *Can stress stop you from getting pregnant.* Retrieved from: www.babymed.com/can-stress-affect-your-fertility-and-stop-you-from-getting-pregnant#:~:text=Stress%20is%20a%20

reaction%20to%20situations%20that%20
can,conceive%2C%20problems%20with%20
infertility%20can%20lead%20to%20stress

Gurevich, R. (2019). *Dealing with fertility treatment
stress.* Retrieved from:
www.verywellfamily.com/fertility-treatment-
stress-1959976

Gurevich, R. (2020). *How much does IVF really cost.*
Retrieved from:
http://www.verywellfamily.com/how-much-
does-ivf-cost-1960212

Gurevich, R. (2020) *12 potential signs you may have
a fertility problem.* Retrieved from:
http://www.verywellfamily.com/symptoms-of-
infertility-1960282

Gutmann, J. (2020). *Transitioning from RE to OB/
GYN.* Retrieved from:
www.resolve.org/support/pregnancy-after-
infertility/transitioning-from-re-to-obgyn/

Gough, B., & Hanna, E. (2017). *It made me feel less
than a man knowing I may never be a dad':
The hidden trauma of male infertility.* Retrieved
from:
www.theconversation.com/it-made-me-feel-less-
of-a-man-knowing-i-may-never-be-a-dad-the-
hidden-trauma-of-male-infertility-84414

Hsieh, C. (2017). *What IVF really feels like.* Retrieved from: www.cosmopolitan.com/sex-love/ a13119206/ivf-treatment-artificial-insemination/

International Surrogate Center. (2020). *Steps during your surrogate journey.* Retrieved from: www.internationalsurrogacycenter.com/steps-to-being-a-surrogate/#:~:text=Surrogate%20 Released%20to%20Personal%20 OB%2FGYN%20Within%20ten%20to,the%20 date%20and%20time%20of%20your%20fir-st%20appointment

IVF Conceptions. (2020). *Surrogacy health insurance covers only surrogacy pregnancy and birthing costs.* Retrieved from: www.ivfconceptions.com/surrogacy-health-insurance/

Long, J. (2017). *How I coped with my wife's infertility: A male's perspective.* Retrieved from: www.drjamielong.com/wifes-infertility-male-perspective/

Martinelli, K. Miscarriage is Common. (2016, October 13). *So why is it such an isolating experience?* Retrieved from: www.washingtonpost.com/news/parenting/ wp/2016/10/13/talking-about-miscarriage-might-be-upsetting-but-we-need-to-do-it/

Mayo Clinic Staff. (2019). *Infertility*. Retrieved from: www.mayoclinic.org/diseases-conditions/ infertility/symptoms-causes/syc-20354317

McFarland Clinic. (2011). *Finding the cause of your infertility*. Retrieved from: www.mcfarlandclinic.com/about-us/news-events/news-releases-34751/finding-the-cause-of-your-infertility

Levine. H. (2020). *How stress can hurt your chances of having a baby*. Retrieved from: www.webmd.com/baby/features/infertility-stress#1

Loma Linda University, Center For Fertility & IVF. (2020). *Types of IVF medication*. Retrieved from: www.lomalindafertility.com/treatments/ivf/ types-of-ivf-medication/

Parents. (2020). *7 Myths about infertility: What's the truth, and what are just old wives' tales?* Retrieved from: www.parents.com/getting-pregnant/infertility/ causes/myths-about-infertility/

Penn Medicine. (2020). *A step-by-step look at the IVF process*. Retrieved from: www.pennmedicine.org/updates/blogs/fertility-blog/2020/april/how-does-the-ivf-process-work

National Health Service (NHS). (2020) *Overview: Infertility.* Retrieved from: www.nhs.uk/conditions/infertility/

NHS. (2020). *Risk factors: Infertility.* Retrieved from: www.nhs.uk/conditions/infertility/

Reimann, M. (2016). "'I was with my wife the entire time.' Polish men's narrative of IVF treatment." *Reproductive Biomedicine and Society, 3,* 120-125. Retrieved from: www.rbmsociety.com/article/S2405-6618(16)30022-3/fulltext

Resolve: *The National Infertility Association.* (2020). Get the facts. Retrieved from: www.resolve.org/infertility-101/what-is-infertility/fast-facts/

Shiel, C.W., MD. (2018). *Medical definition of conception.* Retrieved from: www.medicinenet.com/script/main/art.asp?articlekey=31242

Southern California Reproductive Center. (2016, August 9). *How to cope with emotional stress of IVF.* Retrieved from: www.blog.scrcivf.com/how-to-cope-with-emotional-stress-of-ivf

Stanford Health Care. (2020). *Egg fertilization and embryo transfer*. Retrieved from: www.stanfordhealthcare.org/medical-treatments/a/assisted-reproductive-technologies/procedures/fertilization-transfer.html

The Storks Nest Surrogacy Agency. (2020). *Gestational surrogate compensation*. Retrieved from: www.storksnestagency.com/gestational-surrogate-compensation#:~:text=Gestational%20Surrogate%20Base%20Compensation%3A%20%2435%2C000%3A%20IVF%20Transfer%20And,%28For%20Single%20Child%20Pregnancy%29%28If%20Multiples%2C%20Add%20%24250%29%20%24750

Trigo, A. (2020). *Mindfulness in IVF: How can you help yourself during IVF?* Retrieved from: http://www.myivfanswers.com/video/mindfulness-in-ivf/

West Coast Surrogacy. (2020). *Surrogate mother costs*. 2020. Retrieved from: http://www.westcoastsurrogacy.com/surrogate-program-for-intended-parents/surrogate-mother-cost

2

Win Fertility. (2020). *Supporting your female partner through infertility.* Retrieved from: http://www.winfertility.com/blog/supporting-your-female-partner-through-infertility/

Win Fertility. (2020). *The physical and emotional toll of infertility treatment.* Retrieved from: www.winfertility.com/blog/stress-of-infertility-treatment-ivf/

Ying, L., Har Wu, L., & Yuen Loke, A. (2016). "Gender differences in emotional reactions to in vitro fertilization treatment: A systematic review." *Journal of Assisted Reproduction Genetics;* *33*(2): 167–179. doi:10.1007/s10815-015-0638-4.